Belly Fat Six

Paul Clargaux

Copyright

Belly Fat Six© 2022

ISBN: 9798352892251
Imprint: Independently published

Belly Fat Six©

Paul Clargaux

Contents

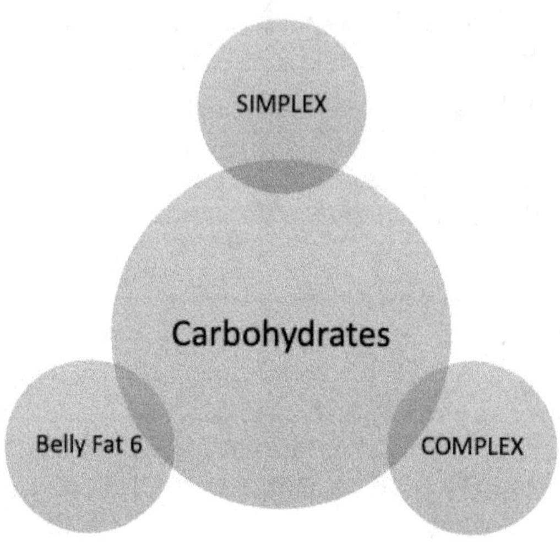

Belly Fat 6 Carbohydrates:

- Sugar
- Alcohol
- Potatoes
- Bread
- Pasta
- Rice

Our Body Constantly Uses Energy

However we consume calories our bodies sort the micro-nutrients required to function, stores some excess and wastes the calories that have no function, cannot be processed, or are exhausted in the functions of our normal daily bodily demands. Waste includes the **Belly Fat Carbohydrates:**

- Sugar
- Alcohol
- Potatoes
- Bread
- Pasta
- Rice

Include processed foods that containing Belly Fat carbohydrates such as burgers and sausages!

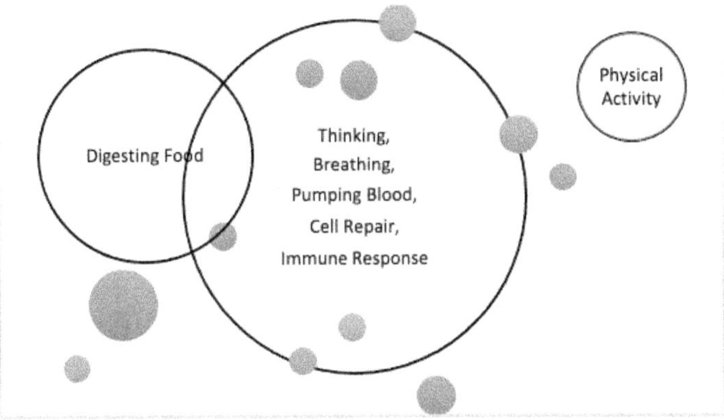

We can help our bodies do less work in avoiding calories that make low to no contribution to our daily performance. So, maintain performance and reduce wasted energy digesting food.

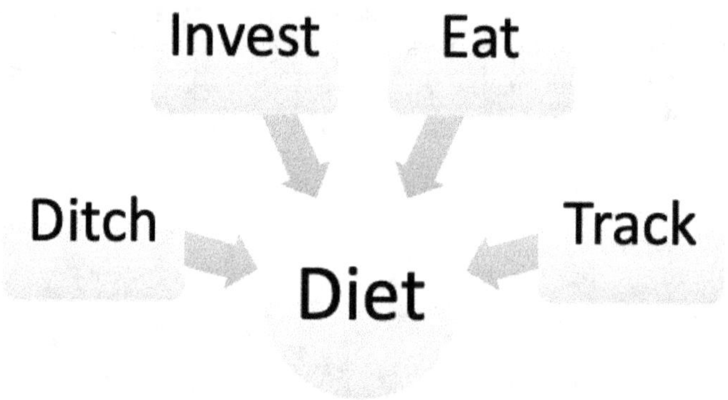

Invest   Eat

Ditch   →   Diet   ←   Track

D.I.E.T.

- D   Ditch Belly Fat Carbohydrates
- I   Invest in YOU
- E   Eat Nutritious Dense Foods
- T   Track your progress daily

I found that there are:

8 Superfoods

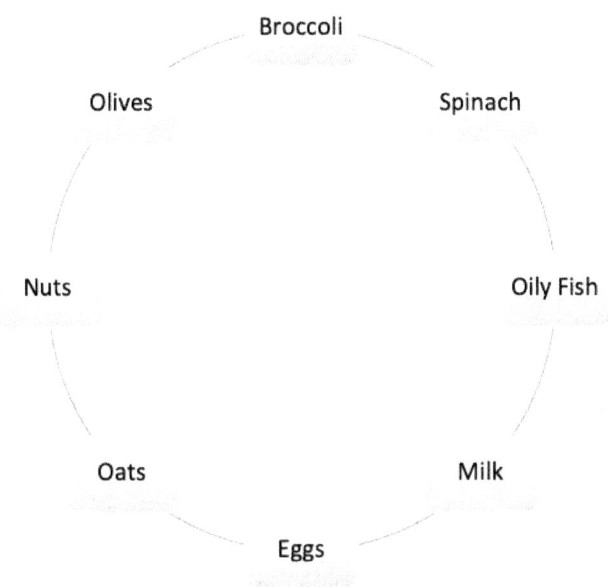

From my research I found that there are things we can control, things we can influence and things we cannot control nor influence!

Clever, Dynamic, Adaptable

Our bodies are 'dynamic and adaptable',

They are smarter than we can ever imagine.

Our hearts pump and our brains think!

Our bodies enjoy being fat.

It's part of our survival mechanism.

Starvation mode.

A bit like storing energy for an unknown future

Therefore, to alter our state,

To change the amount of body fat

To lean body mass,

We must trick our bodies

Into weight loss mode

Ditch the 6 Belly Fat Carbs

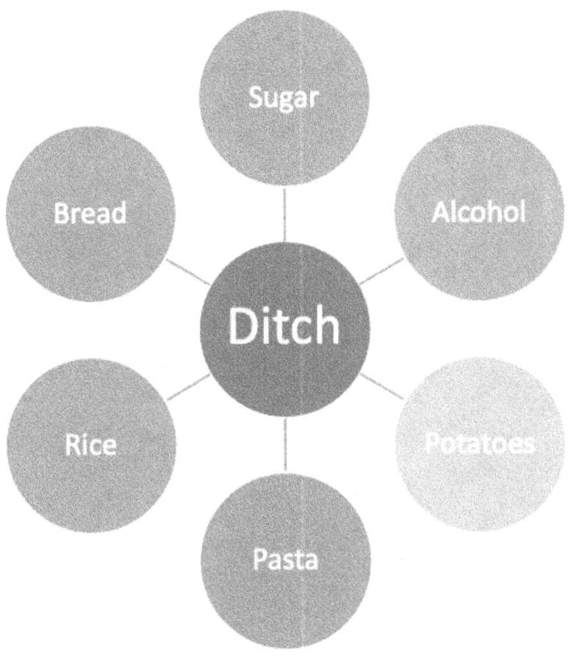

I just want to change, but HOW?

Where Do I Start?

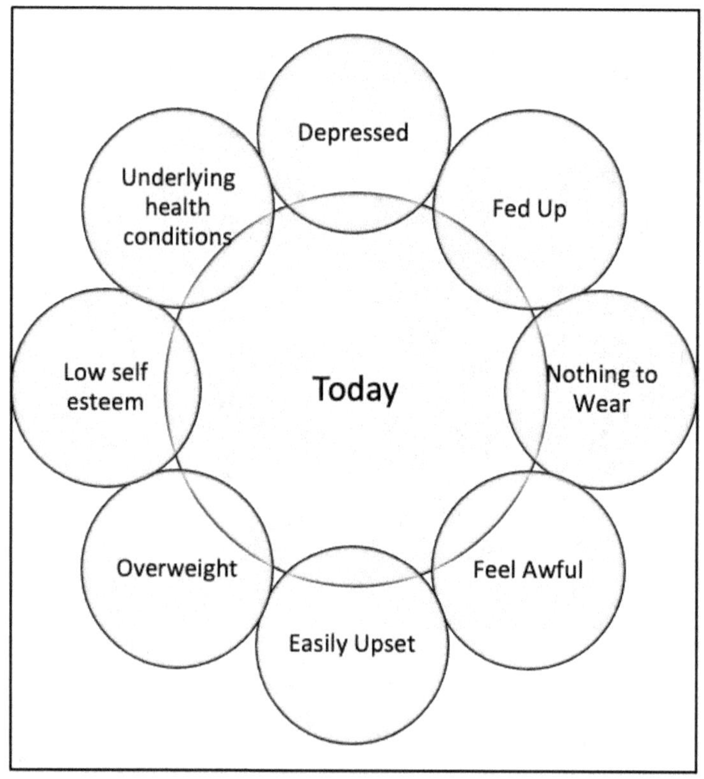

Consult your doctor before starting any weight loss programme.

Ask Questions and challenge the status quo:

The Food Mix

- What do people want from food?
- What do nutritionists want from food?
- What do farmers want from food?
- What do food manufacturers want from food?
- What do Retailers want from food?
- What does Advertising tell us about the food they want us to eat?
- What does the medical profession want from food?
- What does the government want from food?

We will try and find some answers for the many people who are trying to lose weight and be healthy while maneuvering through the ambiguity of the Food Mix. Diet is a mental health issue with many underlying myths and controls, this affects everyone from stay-at-home parents to successful entrepreneurs but dieting failure and entrepreneur failure is rarely regarded as a mental health issue! However, a boxer in a 50/50 win/lose scenario, loses and breaks down and cries and this is a mental health issue.

- How many people cry over not fitting into their clothes?
- Who influences us?

The Food Mix Influencers

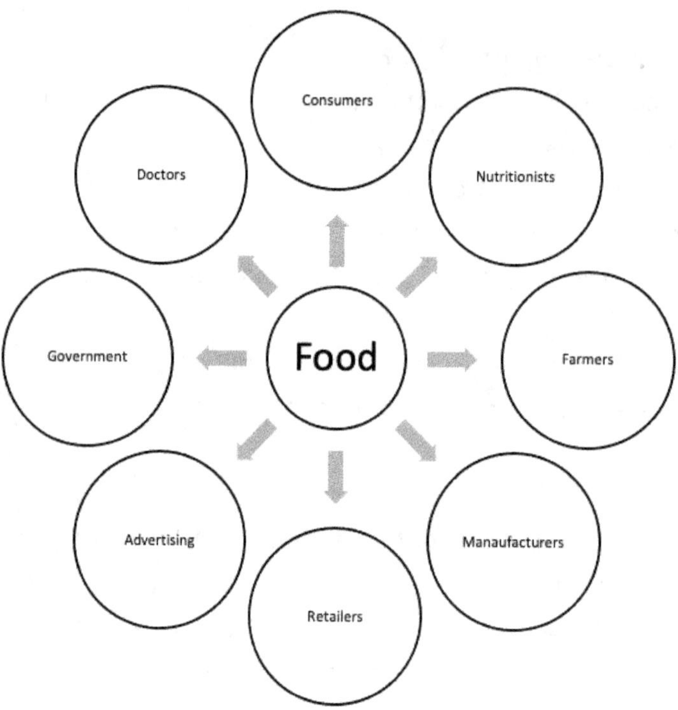

- The influencers.
- Different interests in the food mix.
- How many supporters of health versus interests in profit?
- Where are YOU in the food mix?

We want to change, but how? What are the steps?

7 Steps to Personal Success

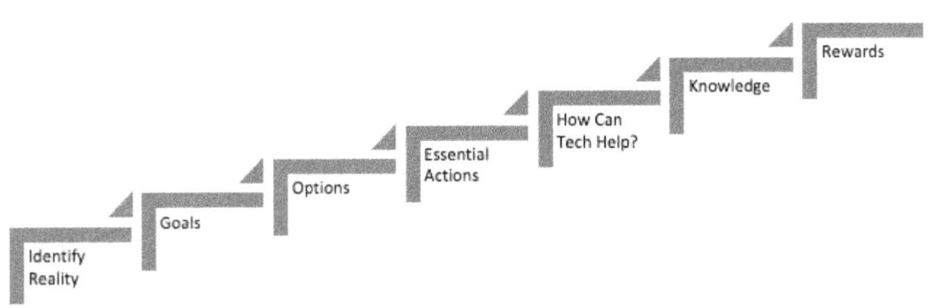

1. Identify Reality. Where are you now
2. Goals. What do you want to achieve and when
3. Options. What are the options open to you?
4. Essential Actions. Decide how you will move from reality to goals.
5. How can tech help? Eg. Apps and a smart watch can help record progress.
6. Knowledge. Records help you understand how to move forward (and backwards)
7. Rewards. How will you view success. Drop sizes, fitter, healthier etc.

Preparation & Actions

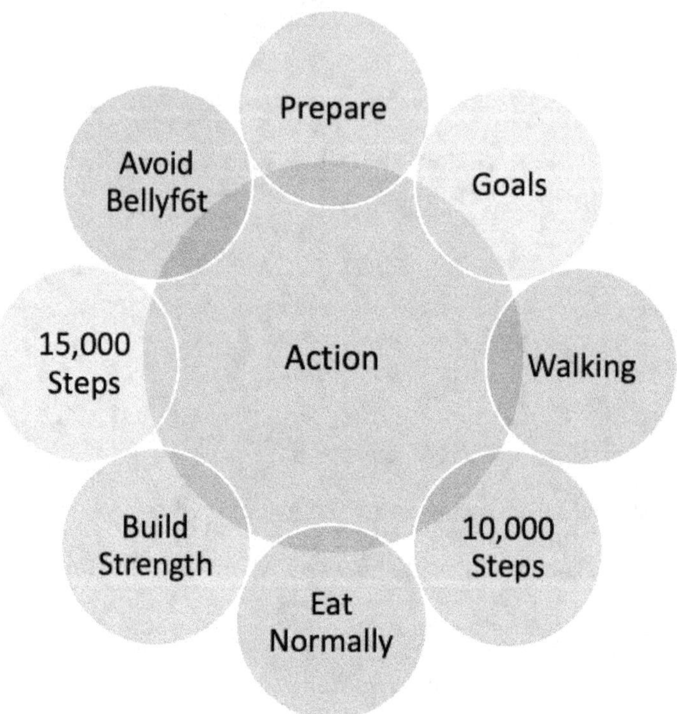

Don't dive in! Carefully consider what we want to achieve for ourselves. Where are we now? What are the things we are dissatisfied with? What would make us more satisfied? These are our goals.

How can we achieve these goals, easily and fast? What are the secrets that will help us make changes that will last for the rest of our lives?

Consult your doctor before starting any weight loss programme.

Work SMART

I found I can maximise my intake of Vitamins and Minerals by focusing on food that contain many of the nutritious elements my body needs.

This means I can ensure vital nutrients while limiting calorific intake meaning my body absorbs more nutrients from less calories. So, this means to me that my body works smarter as there are fewer empty calories to process as waste (to create fat stores)!

I focus on the identified superfoods:
- Milk
- Eggs
- Broccoli
- Spinach
- Nuts
- Oats
- Oily Fish
- Olives
- Cheese

I focus on any foods that provide nutrients in abundance. I have done some of the work for myself and attached charts that highlight identified nutrients to make my food choices easier.

I may choose to eat the foods that are packed with nutrients, or try new foods, or eat the Belly Fat Six, it's entirely my choice! I only advocate to avoid the Belly Fat Six when trying to reduce or control weight.

It's a simple technique:

Focus on vitamins and minerals that our bodies require, abstain from foods that are high in calories but low in nutrients, avoid foods that are caffeine loaded as this deletes the absorption of some nutrients. Also, be careful of foods that provide excess vitamins and minerals as these can have negative effects on mood such as exceeding (rda) vitamin A.

- Vitamins from a Balanced Diet – Vitamin Dense Foods
- Balanced Diet – Mineral Dense Foods

There are two charts below that focus on our food and the vitamins and mineral content. You can use this link to access A4 pdf charts:

https://drive.google.com/drive/folders/1PB97-dcmnSTrVa--ZnD2BNlInA-qv0Be?usp=sharing

Aim for nutrient dense foods and limit calories. In this way we will reduce the work our bodies have to do in processing our food intake.

Vitamins from a Balanced Diet – Vitamin Dense Foods

Vitamins	Broccoli	Leafy Veg	Spinach	Nuts	Oats	Carrots	Peppers	Olives/Oil	Spices	Oranges	Apples	Banana	Oily Fish	Cheese	Milk	Eggs	Poultry	Beef	Lamb	Pork
A	✓		✓			✓		✓					✓	✓	✓	✓				
B1 Thiamin	✓				✓					✓	✓				✓	✓				✓
B2 Riboflavin	✓		✓		✓						✓		✓	✓	✓	✓				
B3 Niacin				✓				✓					✓		✓	✓	✓	✓	✓	✓
Pantothenic Acid	✓				✓										✓	✓	✓			
B6	✓		✓	✓	✓	✓		✓			✓	✓			✓	✓	✓	✓		✓
B7 Biotin						✓														
Folate Folic	✓	✓	✓	✓						✓					✓					
B12													✓	✓	✓	✓		✓	✓	✓
C	✓	✓	✓					✓		✓		✓			✓					
D													✓		✓	✓				
E	✓		✓	✓				✓							✓	✓				
K	✓	✓	✓	✓		✓		✓			✓				✓	✓				
Calcium	✓	✓	✓	✓				✓			✓		✓	✓	✓					
Iodine													✓							
Iron	✓	✓	✓		✓			✓					✓			✓		✓	✓	✓
Total	11	5	9	6	5	4		7		3	5	2	8	4	13	11	3	4	3	5

Note: Milk, Eggs, Broccoli, Spinach, Oily Fish
Vitamin A is also a contributor of depression so caution here, and caffeine should be limited too.

Balanced Diet – Mineral Dense Foods

Minerals	Broccoli	Leafy Veg	Spinach	Nuts	Oats	Carrots	Peppers	Olives/Oil	Spices	Oranges	Apples	Banana	Oily Fish	Cheese	Milk	Eggs	Poultry	Beef	Lamb	Pork
Beta Carotene	✓		✓			✓	✓		✓											
Chromium	✓																			
Cobalt	✓		✓	✓	✓								✓							
Copper			✓	✓	✓			✓				✓				✓				
Magnesium	✓	✓	✓	✓	✓			✓				✓	✓	✓			✓			
Manganese			✓	✓	✓							✓								
Molybdenum	✓		✓	✓	✓															
Phosphorus	✓				✓								✓	✓			✓	✓	✓	✓
Potassium	✓	✓	✓	✓		✓		✓		✓	✓	✓	✓				✓			
Selenium	✓			✓	✓								✓					✓	✓	✓
Salt								✓						✓						
Zinc					✓			✓					✓	✓	✓	✓		✓	✓	✓
Total	8	2	7	7	8	2	1	5	1	1	1	4	6	4	1	2	3	3	3	3

Note: Broccoli, Spinach, Nuts, Oats, Oily Fish, Olives, Cheese

The totals highlight the number of minerals found and not the RDA%

I couldn't lose weight in lockdown at first. And then I did. This is my experience it's for others to decide for themselves if this may be the lifestyle choice for them. The question for me was, what controls our weight and how can we control our lifestyle in an easy understandable way? No jargon and not too much scientific explanation.

What I found through adding data to simple analysis charts was quite remarkable and valuable information. I think it's more than diet and exercise. Well, I think it's mostly our diet, or at least it is for me, as this affects how our bodies function both through the digesting of the type of food, we decide to eat but also how those choice foods affect the thousands and thousands of bodily functions we make daily. Most of our body functions it seems, just happen without us having any conscious control over them!

Body functions like pumping blood and breathing for example, we can influence our breathing by holding our breath admitted but ultimately, our body tells us to breathe deeper or shallower as we exert energy or rest. However, has anyone tried to influence the pumping of blood or the digestion of food? I couldn't imagine how many calories we burn when our heart continuously pumps the blood around our body all-day and every day or the calories we burn when digesting food or even thinking.

Even my dog's vet told me that my dog burns more calories doing tricks and tasks than just running around so the same must be true for us humans too! Well, that's what I thought anyway.

It makes sense to me, that more efficient pumping may be attributed to the better fuels we ingest, that's the more nutrient dense foods the more efficient our diet (inputs) and the better our performance (outputs). Much like buying normal fuel for our cars or buying premium fuel, more miles and a cleaner engine, better maintenance, and performance and maybe that applies to our bodies too.

Good, better, best fuels may mean the same quantity but improved bodily function for example water, green tea or honey and lemon with green tea - is that good, better, best?

Good Better Best (example)

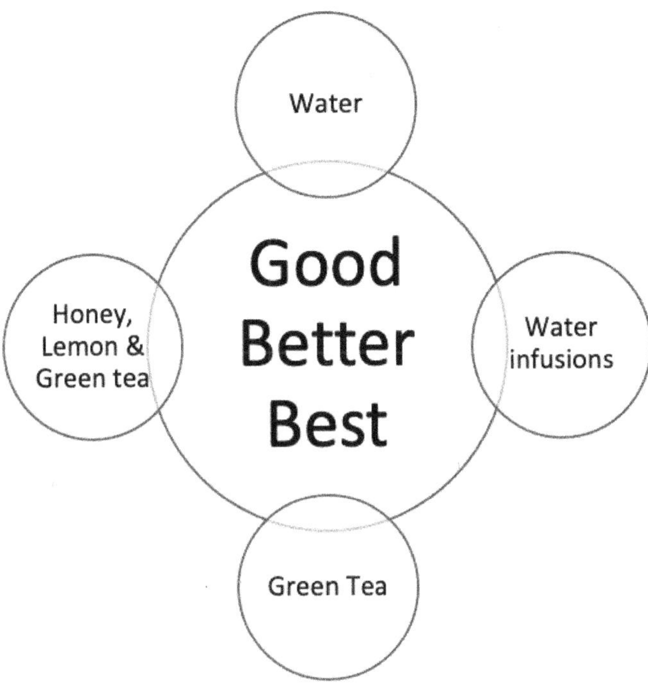

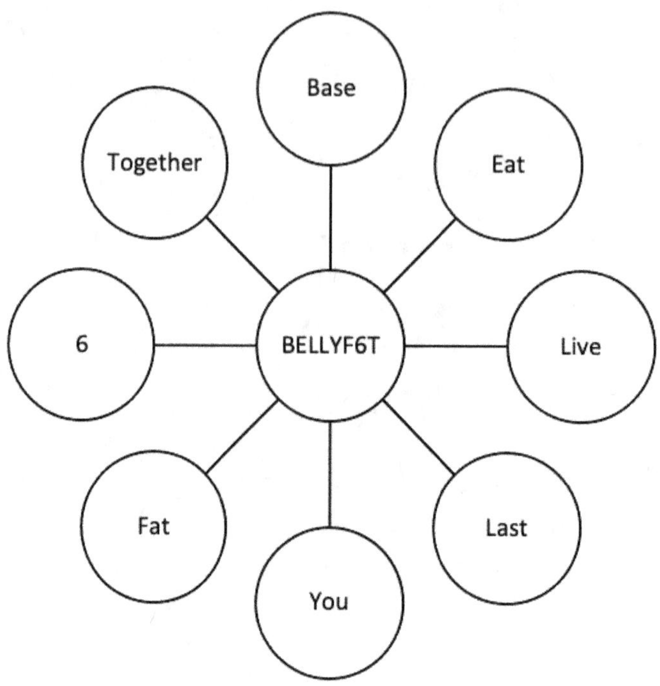

Base	Record your starting point!
Eat	Eat well and change what you eat
Live	Have a fun, healthy life with easy nutrition
Last	An eating system to last your lifetime
You	This is all about you, your diet, your life
Fat	Not all fats are bad, Belly fat is.
6	Don't eat Belly Fat carbs, that's the BellyF6t
Team	We are all in this together, spread the word

Then of course it's what we do with our bodies. Take the vehicle example mentioned above, we have different vehicles for different performance needs, family cars, saloon cars or off-road vehicles all have a different purpose and require different types of fuels and lubricants and vary in delivering suitable performances. There are better fuels for a reason. Premium fuels mean better performance, improved fuel efficiency and less maintenance. If we use the wrong vehicle, the wrong fuel in the wrong terrain then we face the possibility of poor, poorer or bad performance or breakdown. Don't take the wrong turn, stay on track and we won't need to play catch up.

Our cars start as bits of metal, plastic, and rubber. Then they change and become cars. When cars end their usefulness as cars, they are recycled into scrap metal and plastic. Essentially, cars are always metal, plastic and rubber!

Processed meats start as meat, wheat, salt, sugar.
Bread starts as wheat flour, yeast, fat, salt, and sugar.

Use the best performing ingredients and we will have more chance of optimising performance outcomes, however; some ingredients are just destined to perform poorly!

People are the same, ingredients! We have different inputs that mean we are different builds, genders, eat different foods, have a variety of jobs that lead to less or extreme stresses, lead different lifestyles, indulge in sport indoors or outdoors and have varying levels of expertise or basic animal instincts. We do different jobs and enjoy different social or sports activities and our focus on different health and fitness issues changes our ability to perform at different levels from social, amateur to professional. Vocational training at work gets us a better position, more time in the gym helps us to be fitter, healthier, and more toned.

So, what happens when we focus on our diet? My research highlighted certain foods, because of sugar or fat content, affected my ability to control my weight and then to fight off obesity and associated disease. Or the sugar and fat put me at risk of heart attack, stroke, cancers and diabetes and makes me more susceptible to mortality when a virus pandemic challenge me. I found a healthy body, healthy mind, and a robust immune response is key to have a fighting chance of survival. Then I understood that eliminating sugars and certain fats and processed foods can reduce the risk of obesity, disease, and mortality. My question then is what else does the food, exercise and lifestyle choices do for our bodies and our minds, for example those migraines or those days when I feel a little bit under the weather, is it my diet, and is it possible to influence my body to maximise the benefits I can expect and achieve more from better lifestyle choices? So, when we decide to eat 'something' or exclude that 'something' what happens inside our bodies and with the millions of natural uncontrollable functions?

Are there foods we should really be replacing with foods that are much better choices and mean our bodies function much better? Are there superfoods? Surely, superfoods are those more rich or dense in vitamins and minerals, aren't they? What foods provide the most nutrients while limiting the need for quantity? Many people believe this is the case and many diets (Plato, Keto, Mediterranean) focus on good lifestyle choices.

I've added:

- What we eat and what we do.
- What our bodies do with what we eat and what we do!
- Our mind and our choices?
- The food we eat and the type of foods we eat?
- Our movement, normal activity, and our exercise?
- In the BellyF6t I've mixed in simple analysis charts to help reason my actions.
- What to avoid, (maximising success)

What affects weight loss success?

- Knowledge
- Psychology, state of mind
- Planning / Preparation
- Starvation Mode
- Our Body Clock / Circadian Rhythm
- Food, Exercise, Rest
- Others / peer Pressure
- Everyone else is an expert

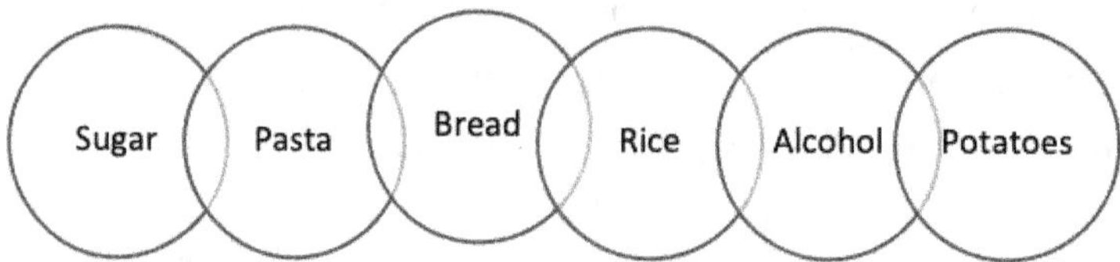

I've found through my management experience that for most humans trying to get anyone to do anything, they don't want to do is mostly impossible. People will only do something when they are ready to do it, when they want to do it or when they need to do it or when the rewards meet their expectations. I think dieting, weight loss and lifestyle change is the same. A doctor telling us to go on a diet, a loved one telling us to lose weight, no matter what the reason, persuasion alone won't move us to action. Don't judge me.

People will only focus on their health and start to diet after we realise that there will be benefits for us in losing weight. Those benefits will vary for everyone, such as attracting a new partner or being healthy or to fit into our loved clothes or the latest fashionable clothes. Whatever the reason for acting it must come from the person requiring change, then we get 'buy in', and that's the most powerful motivator.

Maximise Effort, Leverage, Scale

The rationale is when we know what is causing the problem we can focus on those things and improve our opportunities of success.

- Exclude the things that are holding us back or causing us harm.
- Include the things that promote the achievement of our goals.
- This means we are 'doubling the chances of great results'!

Avoid	Eliminate	Promote Good Mental Health
<ul><li>Too Much Food</li><li>Too Much Bellyf6t</li><li>Too Many Mealtimes</li><li>Too Much Wheat</li><li>Too Much Sugar</li><li>Too Much Stress</li><li>Too Little Exercise</li></ul>	<ul><li>Bacon</li><li>Sausages</li><li>Burgers</li><li>Sweets</li><li>Candy</li><li>Chips</li><li>Cookies</li><li>Crisps</li><li>Frozen Foods</li><li>Ready Meals</li><li>Trans Fats</li><li>Saturated Fats</li><li>Red Meat</li><li>Butter</li><li>Full Fat Dairy</li><li>Baked Foods</li></ul>	<ul><li>Oily Fish</li><li>Beans and Legumes</li><li>Berries</li><li>Leafy Greens</li><li>Water</li><li>Omega 3 Fatty Acids</li><li>B Complex Vitamins</li><li>Vitamin B12</li><li>Folate</li><li>Calcium</li><li>Chromium</li><li>Iodine</li><li>Iron</li><li>Lithium</li><li>Selenium</li><li>Zinc</li></ul>

Whether this is food, exercise, or mental health, we can leverage or results by having knowledge of actions we can take, things or places to avoid and people who can support us. I found that food and the way it is cooked (such as frying) both affected my mood, emotion, stress, and anxiety. **The food that helps promote our required nutrients include: Broccoli, Spinach, Nuts, Oats, Oily Fish, Olives, Cheese, Milk, Eggs**

The vitamins & minerals that promote better mental health.

	Broccoli	Leafy Veg	Spinach	Nuts	Oats	Carrots	Peppers	Olives/Oil	Spices	Oranges	Apples	Banana	Oily Fish	Cheese	Milk	Eggs	Poultry	Beef	Lamb	Pork
B1 Thiamin	✓				✓					✓	✓				✓	✓				✓
B2 Riboflavin	✓		✓		✓						✓		✓	✓	✓	✓				
B3 Niacin				✓				✓					✓		✓	✓	✓	✓	✓	✓
Pantothenic Acid	✓				✓										✓	✓	✓			
B6	✓		✓	✓	✓	✓		✓			✓	✓			✓	✓	✓	✓		✓
B7 Biotin						✓														
Folate Folic	✓	✓	✓	✓						✓					✓					
B12													✓	✓	✓	✓		✓	✓	✓
C	✓	✓	✓					✓		✓		✓			✓					
D													✓		✓	✓				
E	✓		✓	✓				✓							✓	✓				
K	✓	✓	✓	✓		✓		✓			✓				✓	✓				
Calcium	✓	✓	✓	✓				✓			✓		✓	✓	✓					
Iodine													✓							
Iron	✓	✓	✓		✓			✓					✓				✓	✓	✓	✓
Beta Carotene	✓		✓			✓	✓		✓											
Chromium	✓																			
Copper			✓	✓	✓			✓				✓				✓				
Magnesium	✓	✓	✓	✓	✓			✓				✓	✓	✓			✓			
Lithium										✓	✓			✓						
Manganese			✓	✓	✓							✓								
Selenium	✓			✓	✓								✓					✓	✓	✓
Zinc					✓			✓					✓	✓	✓	✓		✓	✓	✓
Omega 3 Fatty Acids													✓							

Less Eating issues and more benefits please!

Eating Issues	BellyF6t	Benefits of Quitting
• Uncontrolled Cravings • Withdrawal Symptoms • Build tolerance to sugar like alcohol and drugs • Sugar product binging	Sugar	• Lose belly fat • Increase energy levels • Improve mental health, mood, clarity, focus, health • Reduce inflammation
• High Glycemic • Impacts Blood Sugar • Raise Insulin • Not good for diabetics • Good for blood pressure, bones, heart health, inflammation, cancer, constipation, skin, immunity, lithium	Potatoes	• Related to weight gain • High carbohydrates • High levels of potassium • Reduce risk of diabetes
• Diabetes • Skin disorder • Inflammation • Raised blood sugar • Increased insulin • Wrinkles	Pasta & Bread (Wheat)	• Reduce risk of Autoimmune disease • Protect Thyroid • Improve weight management • Prevent hypoglycemia • Increased energy • Reduce risk of diabetes • Reduce risk of heart disease • Reduce allergies and asthma
• Raise blood sugar • Constipation • Diabetes • Weight gain • Low nutrition • Allergies • Starchy • Increases Hunger Pangs	White Rice	• Weight loss • Get nutrients from other foods • Less risk of inflammation • Improve skin • Less risk of allergies • Reduce sugar intake • Control Hunger
• Hangover • Memory loss • Lack of focus • Indigestion • Heartburn • Debt • Increased heart rate • High blood pressure • Risk of falls • Personality change • Liver scaring • Cirrhosis of liver • Sepsis • Death • Overweight	Alcohol	• Improved Sleep • Hydration • Reduce Calories • Save Money • Skin improves • Heathier, fitter • Improve Liver Health • Mood improves • Concentration • Better memory • Easier weight loss • Reduce blood pressure • Breathing improves • Stomach feels better • Improved relationships

Having recognised our need for change there is then a shift away from what needs to change to how we can achieve our new desires, that's positive action. This action will depend on a host of things. It will include, time, money, and pain, lots of pain but also the knowledge required for successful outcomes. There are a host of diet plans and many experts and mostly the diets work but we must do them, follow the advice to achieve the results no matter how uncomfortable they make us feel, endure the pain because the gain is worth it. However, many diets involve a lot of hard work and go for a quick fix and eventually the benefits are lost along with the knowledge of the diet. The diet tried and failed disappears until the next fad comes along.

We are sure that dieting requires a change in our attitude of mind as we are going to exclude certain foods and do more activity. However, in this case, the diet, we believe we don't need to work overly hard at limiting food or taking lots of exercise when we work at eating smartly.

Many people are looking for the trick to lose fat and think there is a magic answer and are mostly disillusioned when fat is lost but returns and money spent is lost along with the weight loss and the memory of the fad diet, but my problem was losing weight in the first place. How was I to get in the weight loss zone. I found myself searching for answers.

How our bodies use energy:

Most energy consumed through pumping blood, immune responses and may more thousands and thousands of uncontrollable body functions.

Many people don't lose weight on a diet, and some put weight on. Our bodies can go into starvation mode and the result is that we won't lose weight or at least not very quickly.

Movement

Digestion

Natural Body Functions

There are a few tricks, and they are not well known, and you are about to learn them here.

1. Prepare for success
2. The BellyF6t Base
3. Eat lots of vitamin and mineral dense foods
4. Exclude - The Belly Fat Six
5. Walk

Focus on this technique helped me cut my body's requirement for food variety as I can achieve high nutrition from limited sources. Preparing my mind and my body and walking will help break the circadian rhythm meaning that by excluding The Belly Fat Six and eating foods with high density vitamins and minerals I will be able to exploit the BellyF6t process for maximum gains and weight loss.

So, we need to understand exactly where we are and what our concerns, issues and problems are. Why aren't we happy? What has made us make the solid decision to change and to lose weight? What do we want to achieve and how important it is to succeed. Are there any other possible solutions, can we just remain the same, go to the gym, eat salads for months or take professional dietary advice. All possibilities.

Whatever we decide to do we must be satisfied that it is the right course of action, and we are prepared to see it through.

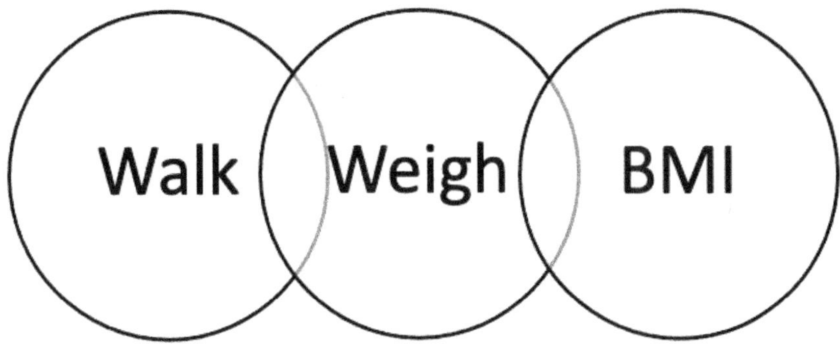

For The Belly Fat Six I weigh daily and calculating my BMI daily too and record the results. There are many apps available that make record keeping easy, but a paper and a pen will do the same job. This helps me stay on track. Other ways to stay on track include help from friends and family or peer groups and gaining knowledge about food, eating less harmful calories, and maximising our intake of nutritious foods.

D.I.E.T.

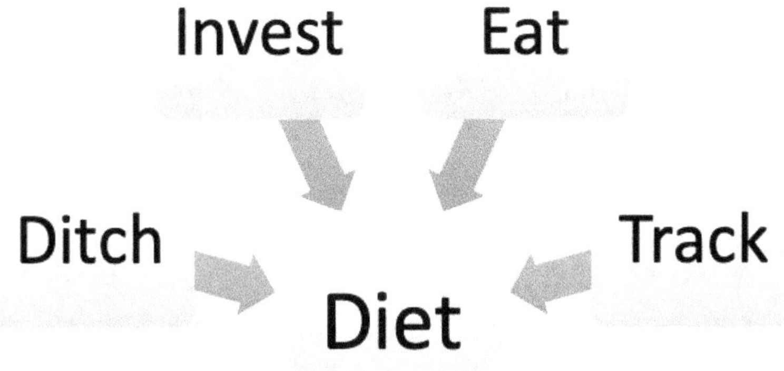

D.I.E.T.

- D   Ditch Belly Fat Carbohydrates
- I   Invest in Me
- E   Eat Nutritious Dense Foods
- T   Track your progress daily

The BellyF6t Larder - Eat or Dispose?

Preparation is the key to success. Planning at work helps us to focus on our goals and this applies to weight loss too, it gets us in the right frame of mind, but unlike people who empty the fridge in the lead up to starting a diet, I didn't want to load excess pounds, and view the start of the diet as an intrusion to my normal day to day life I lead. However, I recognised that the start of a lifestyle change should be celebrated.

Therefore, my Bellyf6t system encouraged me to take time to prepare my body and mind for these most important life changes. For a few weeks ahead of starting I reduced the stores of Belly Fat Six. Being in the best state of mind helps me make better decisions that mean I can take the right actions too.

Also, this means I can break down the technique into two parts, step one mental preparation and step two weight loss. My research found the preparation helps me reset my body clock/circadian rhythm and this meant for me tricking my body to avoid going into starvation mode. Then with adding smarter food sources such as mineral and vitamin rich foods with less calories, weight loss results will be on track and fast. The technique helps us understand how to effect results and to put in place a workable solution I won't forget, a lot like remembering how to ride a bike. I'll never forget how to achieve weight loss results from this lifestyle process. I can control when I want to avoid the Belly Fat carbohydrates. My focus is on nutritious mineral and vitamin dense foods (from less 'Belly Fat Six' carbohydrates).

I quickly realised the benefits of The Belly Fat Six included reduction in obesity and lower BMI without the pain of traditional diets or fad diets and without the need for a heavy workout routine. I had learned a weight loss technique and acquired new knowledge about myself, and that experience has become my lifestyle choice, educated on how to eat less, and control my weight, maintain weight, lose weight, or gain weight. This helps me maintain my lifestyle choices.

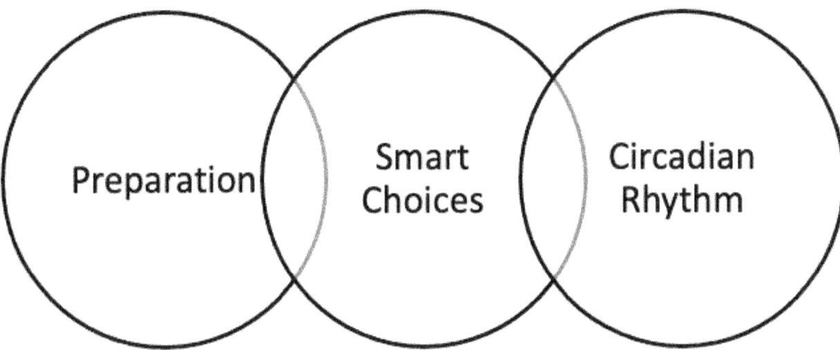

Half the battle is the knowledge, I only find the questions easy when I know the answer. Once I have the 'know how' about my own personal diet management, it becomes as easy as riding a bike and once we know what to do, we never forget. We can connect with new ways of staying in shape and in good health and we can easily 'get back on the bike' when we fall off, we always do, that's life'! In many of life's successes some of it is from luck and much of that success is from the knowledge we already have or gained from our mistakes however, the mistake is making the same mistake over again.

So, I now understand the need to exclude negative foods from my diet. I've also realised I need to ensure my body is nourished with high density foods, 'superfoods', that provide all the vitamins and minerals I need to meet daily demands on my body. However, I've also learned a technique to apply in situations where other dietary needs are highlighted or when things might not go according to plan, when in a pandemic for example, but more on this later!

Finally, I'm not the best at this but keeping records of our successes and failures is also key, I found daily records a great motivator and a massive help. I kept everything simple, using my smart watch and the fitness programme and added my dietary inputs throughout the day. This way I had a running display of my intake and outputs and my achievements. So, I found, there is no real trick it's only a technique that's easy once we know it. My knowledge choices are simple:

1. Prepare for success (to change our habits)
2. Break the BellyF6t Base (Base is our starting point)
3. Eat lots of vitamin and mineral dense foods
4. Exclude the Belly Fat Six
5. Walk

I found and fully believe that everything I do, that everything people do is a process! The process may become habitual (old habits) but it's still a process. The process is simple once we understand it and we get better results the more we refine the process, that's just what we do as people, make things better. And all processes are measurable whether they are tangible or intangible, there's always a way. A great example is our food intake, and our exercise can be measured in weight, volume, distance and converted into calories in and out that reflect in a weight loss or a weight gain and make us feel emotive about our effort. So, many different measures. Change is a process too!

**Physical
Activity**

**Food
Choices**

**Natural Body
Functions**

Therefore, I needed to get to grips with the knowledge that it's down to me to get the results I desire, no-one else will do it for me. My results are determined by my ability and strength to embrace the techniques I developed for me personally.

This required a little preparation and planning, not quite on a military scale. I only needed to change my thought process to alter my daily routines and form new habits. I realised that while, like most people, I don't like change. However, change is inevitable and causes some discomfort at first and then I realise that to achieve better results, I should have been doing the new stuff all along!

So, my new habits, desires and goals must be in line with my planning and preparation, my natural reactions to my body rhythm, my nutritional wants and needs and my choice of positive foods over negative foods.

Then, keeping records of how my new routines affect my body and mind and how I react to my new lifestyle choices will provide the knowledge and information for me to develop further, that's of course, if I feel the need to improve further.

What we focus on matters

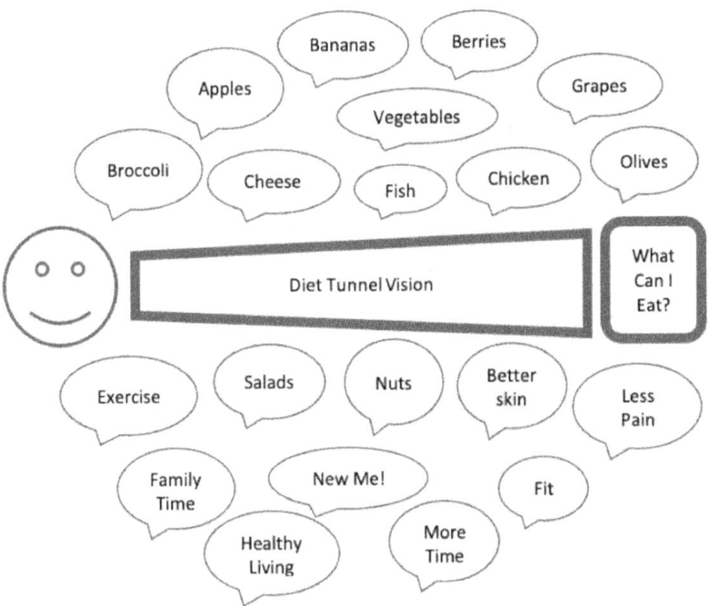

Other things I can do to stay on track:

I thought that I could and should regularly review the foods that are rich in vitamins and minerals and ensure my diets are loaded with nutritious food. Having recently discovered the thymus gland and what this means to health and fighting off disease I changed my routines to include possible thymus health and stimulation. This includes food to encourage health systems for cell development, thymus stimulation, exercise and massage while also noting the importance of keeping warm and how this helps to stop worsening infections.

When trying to change it is very easy to find myself falling back into my old ways particularly if I find myself in in the old familiar circumstances. To avoid these lapses takes a little planning. I spread meals throughout normal waking hours and daylight hours and carry healthy snacks with me. One thing I noticed was the difficulty in eating raw vegetables and salads. I got bored easily. To overcome the boredom and increase enjoyment and consumption I finely chopped raw vegetables and salads. This means the vegetable and salad portions are more dense and easier to eat, while delivering rich levels of vitamins and minerals in the quantities I need. This now means I can eat more of these foods more easily and quickly, staying fuller and more nourished for longer.

A favourite of mine being a small sandwich bag with finely sliced broccoli stalks and carrots and a handful of black olives, simple, nutritious, and healthy, I can carry this with me and snack throughout the day. Then prepare in my mind the daily eating routines.

- Breakfast, Morning snack, (fruit and veg)
- Lunch, Afternoon snack, (fruit and veg)
- Dinner and Evening snack, (fruit and veg)

This ensures I am never hungry for long although to feel hungry at times is purely natural and welcomed (and is a sign we are losing fat stores).

I avoid the Belly Fat Six like the plague. Eating any of these foods will mean I don't lose belly fat and even worse I am adding to what is already there! I will be doing myself a double mis-justice! I find it's always beneficial to plan my meals in advance so that I always have plenty of nutritious food sources available. This helps me to stay on track too. But also shopping trips are more easily planned and this encourages me to stay away from the Belly Fat 6 in the supermarket.

I try and include the 8 Superfoods too, as much as possible. Not easy for everyone who may follow special or strict dietary routines and I may need to supplement some foods for others. Any supplements made are ideally aimed at matching the high mineral and vitamin content as well as excluding The Belly Fat Six.

So now my daily routine focus is something like this:

1. Knowledge - of my body and what I eat
2. State of mind - having a 'can do attitude' to exclude Belly Fat Six
3. Planning - preparing for daily success
4. Starvation Mode - 'my body wants to hang on to my fat'!
5. Body Clock / BellyF6t Base - my body does things itself
6. Food - all foods provide varying amounts of nutrition
7. Belly Fat 6 - avoid the 'Belly Fat carbs'
8. Exercise - in moderation but don't get injured
9. Rest - is the time for our bodies to repair itself
10. Help - support, family, friends, doctors, gym, and research

2 4 6 8	
2 Steps	1. Preparation, Non-diet things 2. Nutrition
4 Activities	1. Increase steps / walk 2. Decide step 2 start date 3. Flexible plans / Calorie count 4. Track Progress. Weigh / BMI
6 Belly Fat 6 Foods To Exclude	1. Sugar 2. Rice 3. Potatoes 4. Bakery (Bread & Pastries) 5. Pasta 6. Alcohol and Sugary Drinks
8 Superfoods Increase these to increase nutrients and reduce calories	1. Broccoli 2. Spinach 3. Oily Fish 4. Milk 5. Eggs 6. Oats 7. Nuts 8. Olives

How My Body Uses Calories

From my research I found our bodies use calories in 3 ways.

1. Natural body functions
2. Digesting food
3. Physical Activity

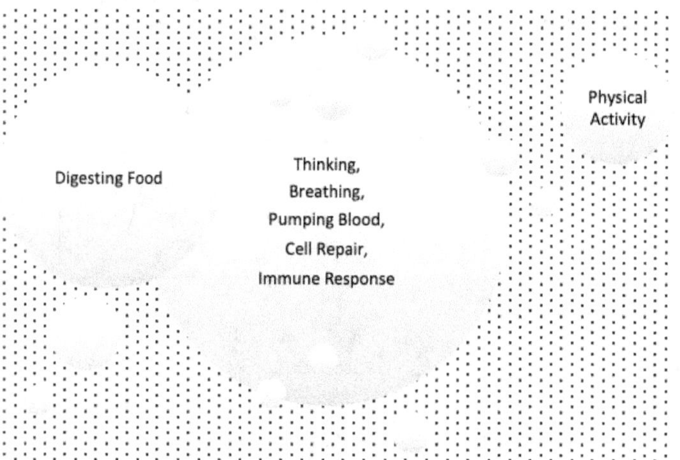

There are thousands of natural daily body functions that are uncontrollable by me! However,

- I believe the BellyF6t, my 8 superfoods and dietary planning may influence the energy spent digesting food (e.g., milk is digested faster than meat. See the BellyF6t Analysis Charts for the difference in nutrition).

- My involuntary movement and my physical activity account for a small amount of my daily calorie burn, and while exercise is important it's not a crucial weight loss activity and breathing, thinking and food digestion probably burn as much or more calories.

The Belly Fat Six

The Belly Fat Six		
Reduce or cut Sugar	Reduce or cut Bread	Reduce or cut Rice
Reduce or cut Pasta	Reduce or cut Potatoes	Reduce or cut Alcohol

Step One	Step Two
<ul><li>Eat a normal daily calorific diet</li><li>Eat nutrient dense foods and the 8 Superfoods</li><li>Start to exclude The Belly Fat Six as much as possible</li><li>Snack on fruit and vegetables</li><li>Walk at least 10,000 to 15,000 steps per day, (not in the kitchen, but outside, around your area,</li><li>Make a route and include hills and flat ground.</li><li>Don't worry about increasing the steps or cutting the time taken. We may lose some weight through activities such as walking but this is about preparing our minds and bodies for success.</li><li>Do this for 4 to 6 weeks (or longer) Until YOU feel ready for step 2</li></ul>	<ul><li>Exclude the Belly Fat Six, eat nutrient dense foods and superfoods</li><li>Maintain your daily walking regime</li><li>Follow the flexible food plan days. Or count calories.</li><li>Pick any plan, any day, in any order.</li><li>If you prefer to count calories use the food lists to a total of a minimum of 1000 to a maximum of 1,500 calories per day.</li><li>Aim for one meal per day</li><li>Snack on fruit and vegetables</li><li>Weigh every day, it doesn't matter what time, weigh yourself and record the result.</li><li>Get to know your body and that your body weight goes up and down.</li><li>Go online and calculate your BMI. It doesn't matter whether we think BMI is a good measure or not, it is a workable aid for this purpose. It helps us maintain focus on our goals.</li></ul>

Without the Belly Fat Six

I found the research shows these six 'simple' carbohydrates all cause belly fat. Without eating these six I should lose belly fat without adding more belly fat! Therefore, **I label them BELLY FAT carbohydrates**. I am making weight loss more difficult if I keep eating the food that causes me to pile on the pounds! The carbs are Belly Fat but so am I if I allow myself to be influenced to eat the Belly Fat Six!

Do my Best:

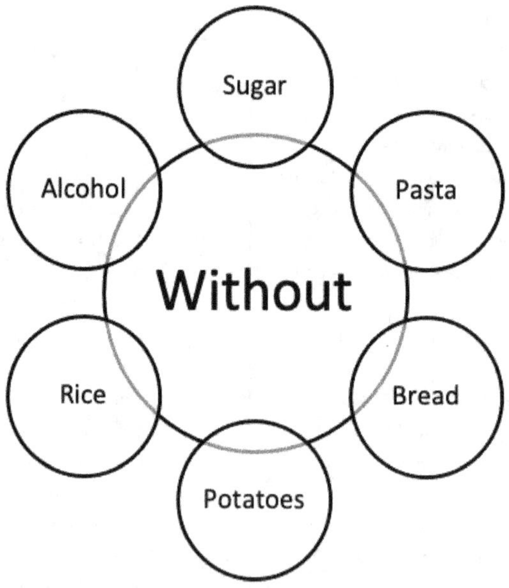

Follow the routine without the Belly Fat 6 for at least 6 Days:

Without: Sugar, Pasta, Bread, Potatoes, Rice, or Alcohol.

Tracking: By using a smart watch and eating programme I found I can control the macro nutrients too and increasing the amount of protein is a proven method of helping to cut fat too.

However, increasing protein as a weight loss tool is a personal choice as this is not for everyone and can bring other health problems.

Day 7 - is my choice. Continue routine or have a break?

The Belly Fat Six Vitamins and Minerals

Note: Almost no beneficial nutrients in any of the Belly Fat 6

Minerals	Bread	Pasta	Rice	Potatoes	Sugar	Alcohol	Vitamins	Bread	Pasta	Rice	Sugar	Potatoes	Alcohol
Beta Carotene	✗	✗	✗	✗	✗	✗	A	✗	✗	✗	✗	✗	✗
Chromium	✗	✗	✗	✗	✗	✗	B1 Thiamin	✗	✗	✗	✗	✗	✗
Cobalt	✗	✓	✗	✗	✗	✗	B2 Riboflavin	✗	✗	✗	✗	✗	✗
Copper	✗	✗	✗	✗	✗	✗	B3 Niacin	✗	✗	✗	✗	✗	✗
Magnesium	✓	✓	✓	✓	✗	✓	Pantothenic Acid	✗	✗	✗	✗	✗	✗
Manganese	✗	✗	✗	✗	✗	✗	B6	✓	✗	✓	✗	✓	✗
Molybdenum	✗	✗	✗	✗	✗	✗	B7 Biotin	✗	✗	✗	✗	✗	✗
Phosphorus	✗	✗	✗	✗	✗	✗	Folate Acid	✗	✗	✗	✗	✗	✗
Potassium	✗	✗	✗	✓	✓	✗	B12	✗	✗	✗	✗	✗	✗
Selenium	✗	✗	✗	✗	✗	✗	C	✗	✗	✗	✗	✗	✗
Salt	✓	✓	✓	✓	✓	✓	D	✗	✗	✗	✗	✗	✗
Zinc	✗	✗	✗	✗	✗	✗	E	✗	✗	✗	✗	✗	✗
Total	2	3	2	3	2	2	K	✗	✗	✗	✗	✗	✗
Carbs %	16	8	9	5	33	1	Calcium	✓	✗	✓	✗	✓	✗
Protein %	20	5	2.7	4	0	1	Iodine	✗	✗	✗	✗	✗	✗
Fat	2	1	0.3	0.1	0	0	Iron	✓	✓	✓	✗	✓	✗
Calories	250	131	130	77	387	43	Total	3	1	3	0	3	0

BellyF6t Analysis Chart 100g examples.

Here are my BELLY FAT carbohydrates! By plotting food v vitamins and minerals I can see these are not very nutritionally dense and are loaded with salt too!

Eating too much of these means being full of negative calories and reduces the chance of achieving the many varied vitamin and minerals required for great health and well-being.

The Belly Fat Six Nutrition Summary

Natural Vitamins and Minerals found in The Belly Fat Six. Note the salt and the lack of variety!

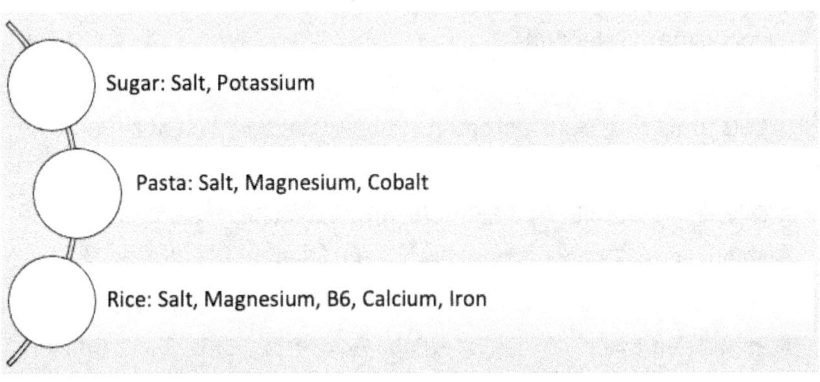

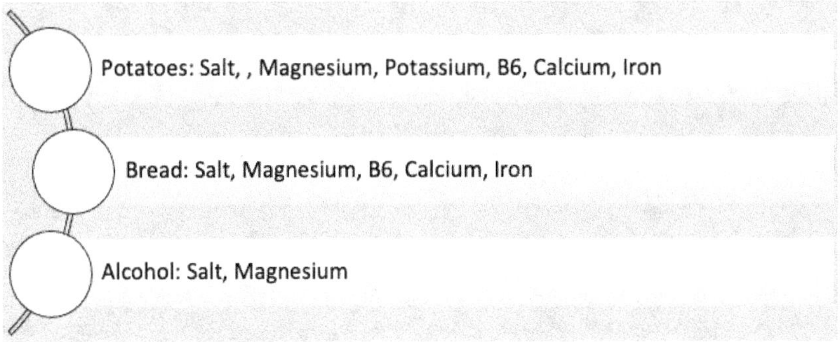

Compare the nutritional value of The Belly Fat Six above with the abundance and variety of minerals and vitamins from the 8 superfoods:

Broccoli, Spinach, Oily Fish, Milk

- Broccoli: Vitamin A, B1, B2 Riboflavin, Pantothenic Acid, B6, Folate/Folic Acid, C, E, K, Calcium, Iron, Beta Carotene, Chromium, Cobalt, Magnesium, Molybdenum, Phosphorous, Potassium, Selenium
- Spinach: Vitamin A, B2 Riboflavin, B6, Folate/Folic Acid, C, E, K, Calcium, Iron, Beta Carotene, Cobalt, Copper, Magnesium, Manganese, Molybdenum, Potassium
- Oily Fish: Vitamin A, B2 Riboflavin, B3 Niacin, B12, Calcium, Magnesium, Phosphorous, Potassium, Selenium, Zinc
- Milk: Vitamin A, B1 Thiamin, B2 Riboflavin, B3 Niacin, Pantothenic Acid, B6, Folate/Folic Acid, B12, C, D, E, K, Calcium, Zinc

Eggs, Oats, Nuts, Olives

- Eggs: Vitamin A, B1 Thiamin, B2 Riboflavin, B3 Niacin, Pantothenic Acid, B6, B12, D, E, K, Iron, Copper, Zinc
- Oats: B1 Thiamin, B2 Riboflavin, Pantothenic Acid, B6, Iron, Cobalt, Copper, Magnesium, Manganese, Molybdenum, Phosphorous, Selenium, Zinc
- Nuts: B3 Niacin, B6, Folate/Folic Acid, E, K, Calcium, Cobalt, Copper, Magnesium, Manganese, Molybdenum, Potassium, Selenium
- Olives: Vitamin A, B3 Niacin, B6, C, E, K, Calcium, Iron, Copper, Magnesium, Potassium, Salt, Zinc

The Yes's v No's

YES - The 8 Superfoods	NO - The Belly Fat 6 (Belly Fat Carbs)
Broccoli	
Spinach	Sugar
Oats	Alcohol
Nuts	Potatoes
Milk	Bread
Eggs	Pasta
Oily Fish	Rice
Olives	

Drinks

I drink as much unsweetened tea, herbal tea, coffee, water that I want or need. (I exclude all sodas including diet drinks or light drinks).

Vegetables

- As many finely chopped raw vegetables or
- As much cooked vegetables that you want:

Broccoli, carrots, asparagus, cauliflower, beetroot, cucumber, cabbage, sprouts, garlic, mushrooms, onions, peppers, radishes, lettuce, spinach, peas, herbs, spices.

Oily Fish

Salmon, sardines, herring, kippers.

Fruit

Apples, bananas, oranges, berries, lemons, limes, grapefruit, papaya, tomatoes, and watermelon etc.

Salad

As much salad as I can eat: Any lettuce, leaves, cabbage, carrots and onions. Add a spoon of dressing or mayo (light) if I wish.

Top Tip: Finely chop the lettuce leaves. This makes it easier to eat and will encourage me to eat more, so I stay full for longer.

Jelly As much Jelly too.

And, I have no issue with honey as there are vital immune properties in honey for healthy cell and thymus such as calcium and phosphorous and zinc too.

Add, my superfoods, Broccoli, Spinach, Oily Fish, Milk, Eggs, Oats, Nuts, Olives. WATER.

Superfoods are Nutrient rich and low in calories. The simple science means our body will spend less resources on digestion and fat storage. I think this is the reason I might occasionally feel tired with no reachable explanation, eating well, feeling well but tired! Why?

Maybe I am exhausting my body with calorific foods that are low in nutrients causing my body to work harder to process waste instead of focusing on the nutrients I could be getting!

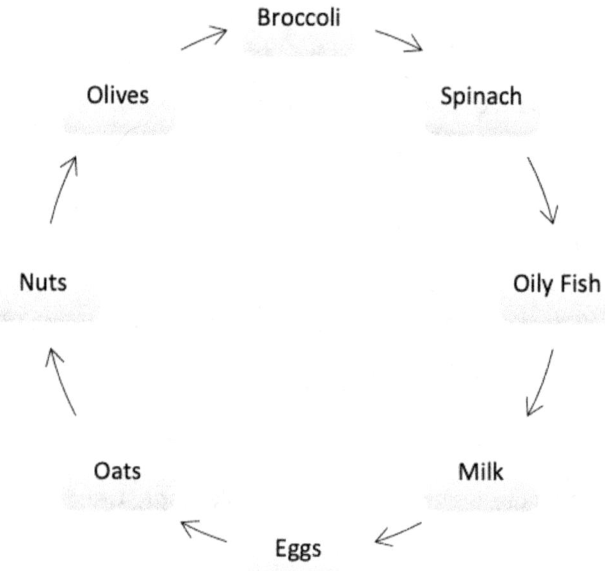

Slave to the Rhythm, Circadian Rhythm

So, our bodies do things that we have no control over, I am a slave. From research I found the circadian rhythm, sometimes known as our body clock or sleep wake cycle. I found that the research suggests what and when I eat affects my metabolism and my well-being and this even includes the time I eat. However, I assume that everything I eat or do, including activity and routines affects the efficiency and regulation of my body clock too. I call this "My Circadian Place" and this is where I am when everything in my body I can't control is in sync. I can influence it (body functions) however, I can't control it. But having regular routines and eating better fuels means my body operates more efficiently and doesn't waste energy processing the Belly Fat Six.

Circadian Rhythm (body Clock, sleep/wake cycle) is the natural processes that happen in my body over every 24-hour period.

Affects: Sleep, Body Temperature, Hormones, Appetite, other body functions and arguably our bodies decision to use fat storage for energy.

My research found extreme issues that contribute to health such as: obesity, diabetes, depression, bipolar disorder, seasonal affective disorder, sleep disorders (insomnia), immune response etc.

Factors Affecting Circadian Rhythm:

- Waking
- Sleeping
- Thirst
- Hunger
- Craving Belly Fat carbs
- Body Functions
- Stress
- Processing food
- Providing nutrients
- Storing fat
- Expressing waste food and water

Other factors include:

- Environment (noise, heat, light, smells, dust, chemicals, toxins),
- medications, work (people/tasks),
- stress,
- alcohol,
- substances,
- poor health,
- anxiety,
- trauma,
- poor diet,
- lack of water,
- low exercise regimes,
- lack of routines,
- relationships,
- injuries.

So, from circadian rhythm I learned my metabolism is based on thousands of uncontrollable bodily functions every day. I assume my body clock or circadian rhythm is just about eating, sleeping, and waking at certain times but this assumption does not account for the millions of other possibilities that can occur and affect my health such as how my body processes the calories, I force upon it.

I ask, what would 'my circadian body' prefer I ate if it could choose? Probably not what my brain thinks, not the Belly Fat Six! It seems despite years of research regarding nutrition that humans are only beginning to explore and uncover the mechanics of our metabolisms, our nutrition, and its affects. However, we seem to know much about marketing BELLY FAT carbohydrates to unsuspecting consumers and this is an economic choice rather than a humanitarian task.

For me diet includes food cravings or BellyF6t Deviancies, the desire for water through thirst and hunger or the need for rewards such as alcohol or chocolate.

- What we eat
- (When we don't eat)
- **How we influence body functions** (not control)
- When we eat

Mind Games

I found research that supports when I diet my body loses weight in the form of fat and chemicals such as leptins. The research suggests that my body then tries to trick me to replace the losses from ceasing my old habits of eating the Belly Fat Six. This seems to be because my body is used to performing the function of storing fats. My body is doing less but doesn't know it yet. But it wants to resist the change imposed upon it. This creates tension between the circadian rhythm and the change in nutrition.

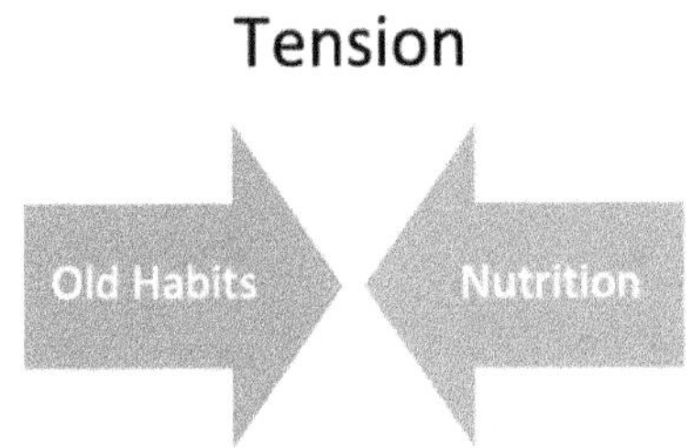

So, I start to crave fatty foods and the Belly Fat Six that will replace the chemicals my brain seems to think that I have lost. I found that when I overcome these rogue feelings my weight loss became easier, more permanent, and habitual.

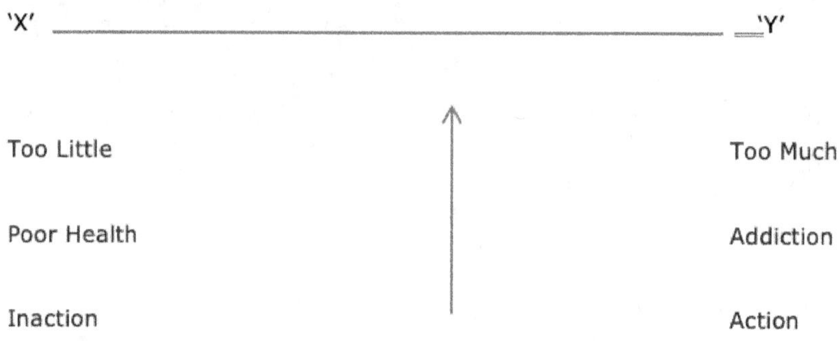

Aim for some action but not too much.

The cravings that I experience when change my diet are pulling me back to my old ways of eating as my body and my mind are in conflict and are clawing back the old me. I want to change but there is tension and therefore, I label the cravings that I desire my Belly Fat Deviants.

BellyF6T Deviances

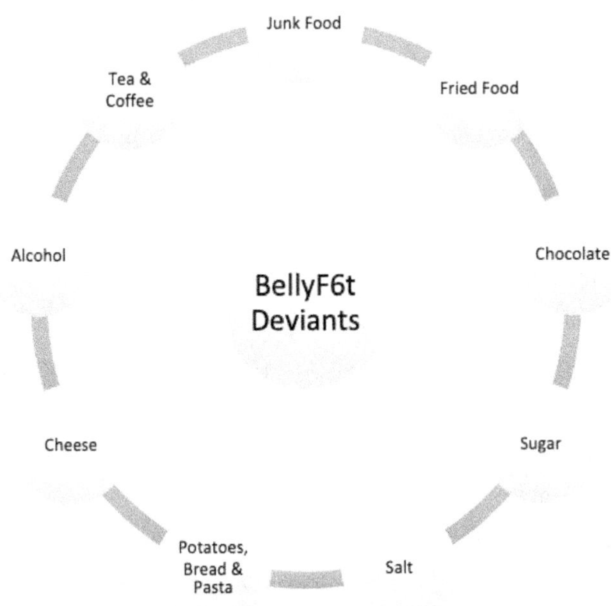

Circadian Rhythm & Food Cravings

I always think I should listen to my body. If I am craving something it may mean my 'body' needs it and my 'mind' needs to feel satisfied. So, I think that craving food types such as the BellyF6t may mean my body and my mental health, and my circadian rhythm is deficient in some way.

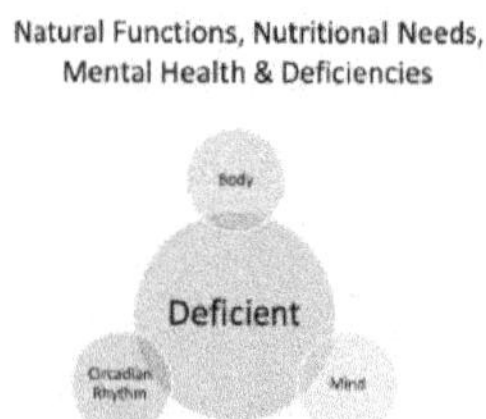

This may be just a change of habit or as I found nutritionists state that this is because of a leptin deficiency! It probably is. The research provides that nutritionists will advise us about the scientific change because of leptins. Going on a diet is a lifestyle change so we should expect cravings for the old ways that we used to live as our bodies don't want to change, however, I recognise that my old ways is the trigger for change. I find if I crave something then I eat it, and move on, no supplements or fake foods, I eat what I crave and satisfy the craving.

I found the best strategy for me to reduce food cravings is by eating nutritious foods that are good sources of nutrients. My 8 superfoods are packed with vitamins and minerals meaning I reduce energy expenditure on processing them, and I found eating these 8 superfoods help provide my body with the nutrients required for my body, help reduce food cravings and avoid the reaching out for any of the Belly Fat 6.

The 8 Superfoods	The Belly Fat 6
Broccoli	
Spinach	Sugar
Oats	Alcohol
Nuts	Potatoes
Milk	Bread
Eggs	Pasta
Oily Fish	Rice
Olives	

So, I think the more I am in sync with my circadian rhythm then the less likely I will have food cravings. Further, 'including' the 8 superfoods while 'excluding' the Belly Fat 6 helps me achieve the harmony I desire. So, I make 'harmony' the craving and not sugary snacks! I found hunger just goes away after a few days of avoiding the Belly Fat carbs and avoiding processed foods is way more natural and healthier.

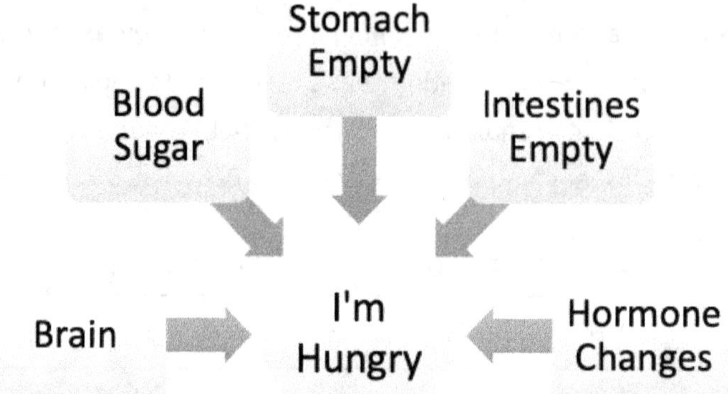

Stomach Empty
Blood Sugar
Intestines Empty
Brain
I'm Hungry
Hormone Changes

Circadian Rhythm and Hunger

I found my hunger is part of the Circadian Rhythm given I can't control my body's signals. However, this is also a sign that my body needs fuel. The body will seek fuel from fat stores if we don't eat, therefore, we must be hungry to lose the fat stores!

When we feel hungry this is a sign that our body needs nutrition. This can be vitamins and minerals rather than calories; however, these cravings will almost certainly drive us to the fridge door and Belly Fat 6! But the hunger pangs are also representative that our bodies will turn to fat stores! As such, I see hunger pangs as a warning that our fat stores are about to be used to supplement the shortage of food intake. I also think this warning is about the quality of the fat stores in providing the nutrition my body needs. For example, didn't my body prefer to store the calories as fat rather than utilise these? Does this mean the stored fat will not provide the nutrition my body requires? However, I do know that using fat stores means I will begin to lose weight. I also, found that after a few days of calorie reduction that the feeling of hunger stopped. Eventually disappearing and replaced with the feeling that I had control over my diet, my nutrition, and my food choices.

So, I must be hungry as that's when
my body decides to use my food stores, my fats!
However, I must eat nutritional dense foods
This ensures my body is not nutritionally denied

When we reduce our calorific intake, our bodies do not suffer the lack of energy resources when we are carrying food stores. Our body will replace the lack of calorific intake from our fat stores. That's just what we think isn't it? The secret is the trigger that makes this happen is our hunger pangs and our understanding of what this means to us and our diets. The hunger pangs and bloating subside.

Controlling the effects of hunger means eating foods that keep us feeling full for longer as empty stomach and empty intestines will signal our brains that we need to be eating. Some people turn to protein as this keeps away the hunger pangs, I prefer my 8 superfoods. However, there are many healthy alternatives for the Belly Fat Six. Preparing healthy snacks helps me control cravings and this can keep me on track when I am trying to exclude the foods that contribute to ill health and weight gain, specifically the Belly Fat 6. So, by being prepared with a constant supply of healthy nutritionally dense foods (fruit and vegetables) I can help my brain think I am not hungry or deficient in any nutrients.

Therefore, excluding the Belly Fat carbohydrates, junk foods and empty calories from my habitual eating routines and adding copious amounts of nutrient rich food, the 8 superfoods, I can trick my brain that there is plenty of food available, I am nourished, full, and to start reducing Belly Fat.

I think food cravings are a momentary feeling they quickly pass and the longer and more often I space out my meals the more my body will get use to my new routines and cease the hunger pangs! I reach for superfood, not junk food alternatives that cost time, money, £pounds.

I found that eating as much as I wanted from fruit and vegetables throughout the day provided me with an answer to hunger pangs while providing me with substantial amounts of vitamins and minerals.

- If I wasn't hungry at the end of the day, I would eat a bowl of cereals or a sardine salad as a last meal before bedtime.
- If I was feeling hungry at the end of the day meal around 1200 calories was sufficient to satisfy hunger.

While it's advocated to skip the bread or the wheat for maximum benefits sometimes a little helps digestion. I monitor the effects and adjust my diet accordingly. Monitoring is a key dietary activity.

I found the main aim is to satisfy my body's vitamin and mineral RDA's (recommended daily allowances) rather than focus on calories, and then my fat stores will make good any calorific deficit. That's my interpretation of the Circadian Rhythm! I can't control this, only influence.

BellyF6t Deviant Triggers

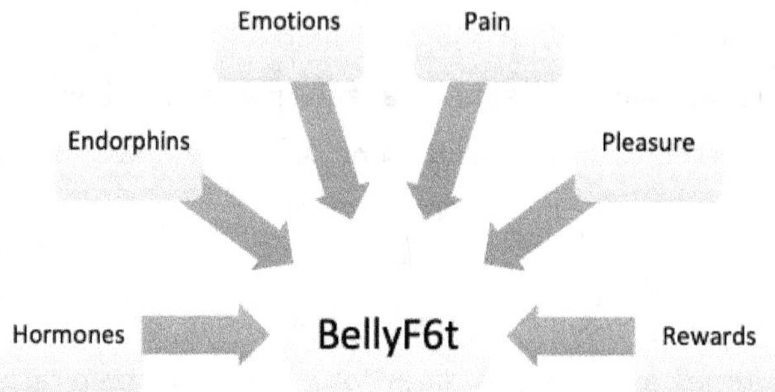

We can avoid BellyF6t by first being aware of them and that we will experience a 'wanting' at some time throughout the day. Plan to avoid dipping into old habits by creating new habits and accepting these are Belly Fat carbs. Look for diets that avoid the Belly Fat Six too. The Belly Fat Six is not a diet in the strict sense as I am focused on avoiding certain foods.

- Go for walks
- Change the routes
- Avoid junk food aisles
- Avoid junk food restaurants
- Prepare healthy snacks and take these with you to work or on your walks
- Practice stress busting techniques, meditate or mindfulness or breathing
- Drink water, carry water with you

Fighting BellyF6t

Some other actions I considered to avoid losing track of my goals.

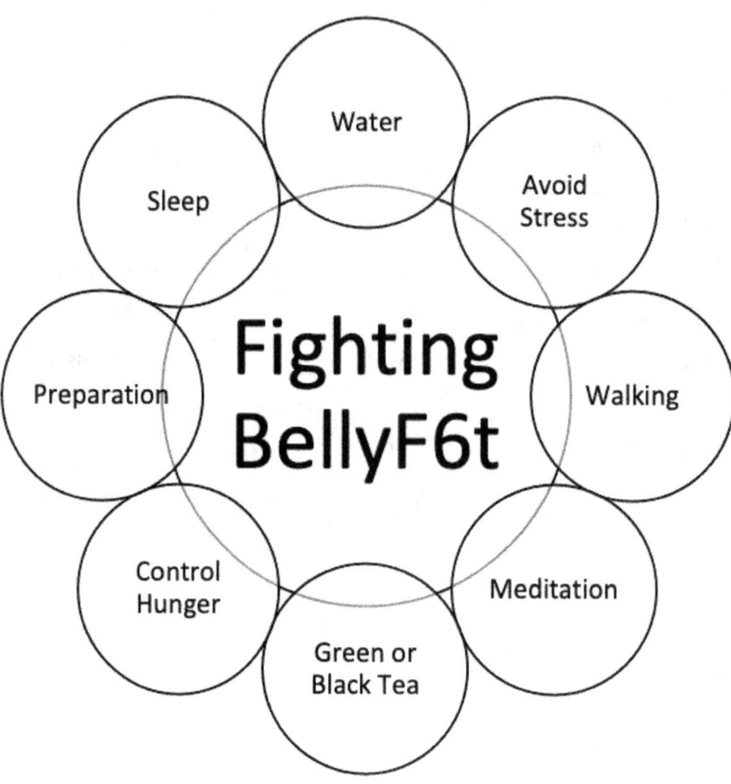

When To Eat

My question is who came up with all these different mealtimes?

- Breakfast
- Morning Coffee
- Brunch
- Lunch
- High Tea
- Dinner
- Supper
- Snacks

One answer is that to sell products it is easier when we instill food norms in people's minds!

- Food producers
- Manufacturers
- Suppliers
- Retailers
- Shops, Supermarkets
- Restaurants
- Cafes

I most probably only need to eat once per day! If I get my nutrients when I eat and how much I eat doesn't matter, surely! One study found that eating all meals within a 10 hour timeframe gave our body time to rest from digestion and I think this is a good point when considering my circadian rhythm too.

1. RECOMMENDED DAILY ALLOWANCE (One meal per day)

Ensure all my daily allowances, my vitamins and minerals are included in this one balanced meal.

Hunger pangs experienced throughout the day, can be set aside by eating as much fruit and vegetables as I want.

Belly Fat Six Deviancy

BellyF6t	Is it Justified?	Think Smart
Salt	Normally a preferred taste or habit.	Avoid. Eat my simplex carbs, raw broccoli, carrots, and olives.
Sugar	Blood sugar deficit, skin tags, diabetes, tooth decay	I take warm milk and honey every night, and this also helps me sleep
Chocolate	Blood sugar, emotional wreck, psychological, stress, taste and feeling	Dark chocolate is better. Crave it, eat it then focus on the 8 superfoods.
Potatoes, Bread, Pasta	Low blood sugar	Finely chopped and sliced broccoli stalks. Vegetable soup.
Cheese	Hungry	Eat cheese with any of the 8 superfoods
Tea & Coffee	Caffeine Addiction Dehydration	Drink water, green tea, naturally squeezed juice.
Fried Chips, Eggs, Burgers, Sausages, Doughnuts, Anything Battered (Fish, Meat)	Food type deprivation Psychological/emotion	Avoid. Find healthy alternatives such as the 8 superfoods
Meat	Iron Deficiency	Eat meat with the 8 superfoods
Alcohol	Reward, Stress	If you must. Remember alcohol is a Belly Fat carb.

Belly Fat Harmony

The Belly Fat Harmony is where I believe I arrive at when all my bodily functions are in tune. Where I am providing all the nutrients my body requires is included here too. My circadian rhythm includes the body clock, hunger, thirst, waking and sleeping and other uncontrollable functions such as cell repair, immune response, pumping blood and semi-thoughts such as food cravings and hunger pangs. I ask, where am I in this myriad of orchestral rhythms?

Part of our body's survival mechanism is believed to be the storage of energy in the form of fat. The body is often assumed to be storing fat from excess foods and from Belly Fat carbohydrates or processed foods, burgers, sausages, and processed meats and from sugar, wheat, bread, and pasta for our future energy needs in times of forced famine. However, there is no calorific value in the fats stored from Belly Fat Six! Therefore, my fat stores are surely nutritionally deficient if based on poor quality food sources.

My research and practical experience found that by preparing my mind and body in advance of any change I can assist the body's natural rhythm and its response to a change in diet and exercise with the result that I begin to lose weight.

I really want to change, my mind tells me I am unfit or unhealthy, but my body craves my old eating habits. I found by eating my normal calorific diet, exercising, and building routines around sleep, mealtimes, work and rest I can harmonise my body clock over a short period. Taking time to prepare for a lifestyle change helps me research and understand the process of change that I am about to focus on to change my lifestyle. It's a choice. Being in the right mindset is 99% of winning, (if you think you will fail you already have).

My body harmonises the body clock or what is known as the natural circadian rhythm because I am, eating healthy, mentally prepared, have routines and therefore, conducting the orchestra for a life of rhythm.

Therefore, I think I begin by changing my lifestyle in a very subtle way. Eat normal calorie in-take and start to exclude The Belly Fat Six and increase activity for a week or weeks to suit my lifestyle. I walk a few miles per day, a couple of miles in the morning and a couple more in the evening, build it into a routine but walk outside, up, and down hills.

How I use energy

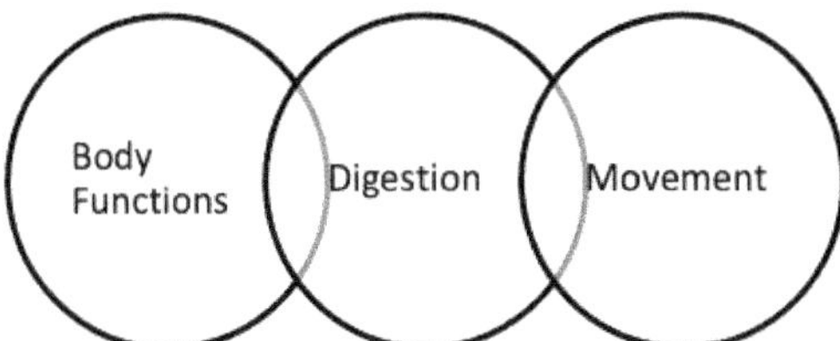

For me, I think it's important that I do not reduce my calories during this harmonising period. I am training my body to be used to a certain amount of exercise and a regular amount of food. My calorie intake will be decided by my natural rhythm and calories used. As mentioned above, in essence, I am preparing my body and mind.

So, initially, I found it's about my mindset, we will do a little more and eat a normal adult calorific intake and try to exclude The Belly Fat Six. Don't diet during this period but consume a normal quantity of calories. Walk, Walk and Walk a few miles a day. I focus on gradual change. and excluding the Belly Fat Six. Mostly, focus on excluding the Belly Fay Six.

When I feel ready, then cut calories. Snack on fruit and vegetables and exclude the Belly Fat Six. I aim for around 1000 to 1500 calories per day of nutritious food. This is the famine my body has been preparing fat stores for. My body, therefore, will make up the deficit by using my stored calories. The result for me was that I began to lose weight. Initial hunger pangs subside after a few days as it seems our bodies become content with a stable intake of calories and the regular burning of calories throughout the day.

Goals

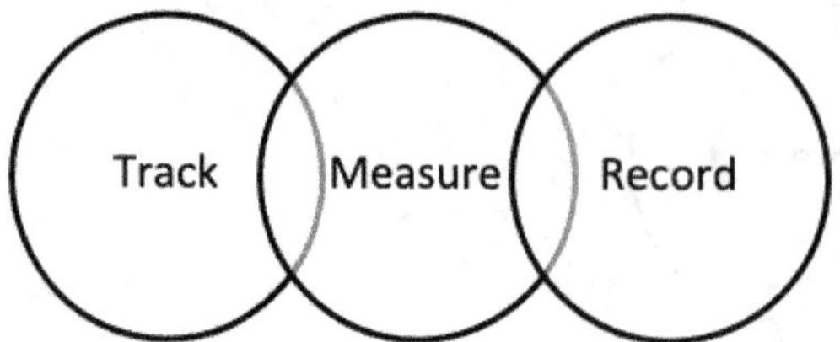

I measure progress as often as possible. There may be a small variation in calories in and out however, our bodies adapt and become comfortable in our new environment. Now the trick I found is to maintain routine where my body burns a lot of calories per day but to reduce the intake to a 1000 or 1500 calories per day and thereby create a calorific deficit.

However, I maintain nutrient dense foods to ensure I am maximising my body's energy requirements but reducing wasted calories that end up exhausting our bodies as we process waste for no apparent reason and the empty calories stored provide no benefit. For example, there is no nutrient basis for eating sugar and salt, and this means our bodies, needlessly, waste energy processing these calories.

Change

As my body is used to (x) calories per day I maintain activity levels and I will continue to use the same (x) calories daily because my body is in a routine, and it wants to maintain the stability of its circadian rhythm.

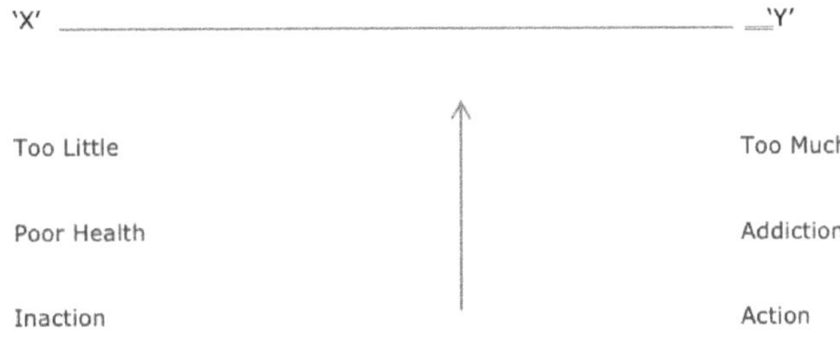

Aim for some action but not too much.

However, as I limit my calorie intake and eat nutrient dense food I'm creating a deficit between calories in and calories out, so I will lose weight.

Body Responses to Change

Normal Rhythm v Disrupted Rhythm	
Normal	**Disrupted**
Caught up on sleep Healthy diet Routine eating times Access to daylight	Sleep deprivation / Jet lag Fast Foods Medications Shift work Stress
Maximise Weight loss Increase endurance Reduce risk of type 2 diabetes Lower blood pressure	Hunger and sugar cravings Disrupts insulin levels Displaced circadian rhythm Poor health choices

When To Eat?

I think the only rule is to eat when I'm awake. In other words, there are no rules. I found that some people eat throughout the day, others eat once per day, some eat breakfast, and some don't and as a result some people are healthy, and others are not. I think if I don't overeat and that I do provide my body with nutritionally dense food that it doesn't matter when I eat. Eating once per day works for me and snacking when hungry on prepared fruit and vegetables keeps the hunger pangs away while providing the nutrients I require. The research I reviewed provides that sleep deprivation is damaging to the circadian rhythm. Sleep affects the body and regulates hunger: Two hormones, ghrelin and leptin stimulate appetite and suppresses appetite respectively. A disrupted body clock can lead to increased hunger and sugar craving, so I aim for 6 to 8 hours sleep per night and eat through the day.

To suppress hunger, I eat protein, fish, meat, chicken, eggs and vegetables and fruits and yoghurt and cheese as these affect leptin levels. I avoid sugar and other sugar derived foods. However, while I eat meat and fish, I now limit the meat and look for vegetarian alternatives.

A nutritious meal I enjoy is a broccoli and salmon omelette that provides most of the daily essential nutrients I need. These 3 foods contain varying amounts of almost **all** the vitamins and minerals I need.

Morning	Evening	Circadian Rhythm
In the morning, in response to body functions, daylight and food, insulin sensitivity increases and melatonin decreases. We feel alive! Energised!	In the evening, melatonin levels rise. Insulin sensitivity decreases. Body is preparing for rest and cell repair. We feel tired.	Circadian rhythm alignment may help maximize weight loss, improve endurance, reduce the risk of type 2 diabetes and lower blood pressure, among other things.

I snack on fruit and vegetables throughout the day to suppress hunger and provide my body with many of the nutrients required for healthy body functions and aim for one substantial meal per day in the evening.

- Blueberries
- Strawberries
- Plums
- Peaches
- Bananas
- Melon
- Carrots
- Broccoli stalks
- Water
- Coffee

I find this works for me but only from my personal research of my own lifestyle. Any changes you may make should be based on the same level of monitoring of what you eat and do but based on the scientific evidence you can find here or through other resources available. Including your own doctor.

The BellyF6T Body Reset

BellyF6t - Body Clock Reset									
	Insulin	Leptin	Ghrelin	Cortisol	Estrogen	Neuropeptide	Glucagon	Cholectokinin	Peptide
Cut Sugar	X	X	X						
Cut Belly Fat Carbs	X	X							X
No Sugary Drinks	X	X							
Balanced Diet				✓					
Fibre					✓	✓		✓	✓
Cruciferous veg					✓				
Protein	✓					✓	✓	✓	✓
Oily Fish	✓	✓					✓	✓	
Magnesium	✓								
Green Tea	✓								
Probiotics							✓		
Walk	✓	✓			✓				
Sleep		✓		✓					
Don't Fast	✓					✓			
Meditate				✓					
Flax seeds					✓				
Music				✓					

The Belly Fat Six - Example Preparation to Start

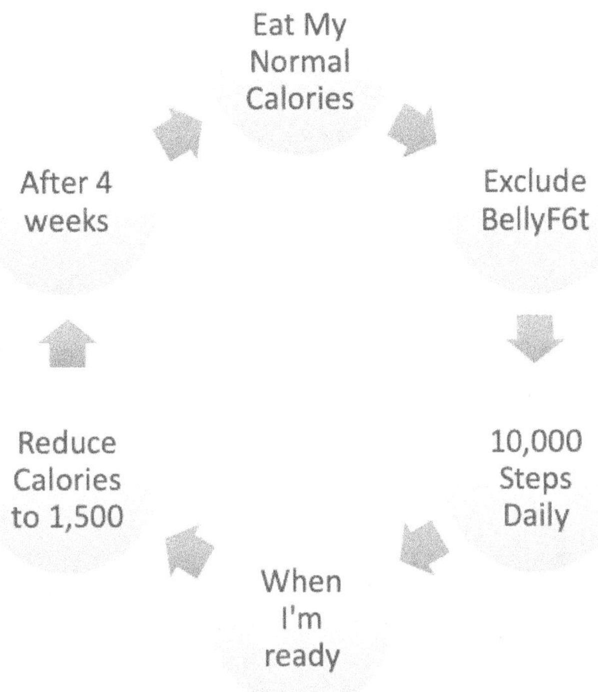

I am preparing mind and body during the first stage of The Belly Fat Six so I can all start from, a reset body clock. Starting point is Circadian Rhythm in balance / equilibrium.

I eat normally initially but exclude The Belly Fat Six whenever possible. All I needed to do was to build a routine so, my mind and body is focused on my well-being. During the first few weeks or I added in a little gentle exercise to encourage routine into my daily plans.

I reduced my calorie intake to around 1200 to 1500 calories per day, continued walking. I increased the high-density vitamin and mineral foods from the tables below. Just by excluding the Belly Fay Six I found I can significantly reduce my calorific intake as the Belly Fat Six are calorific intense while nutritionally negative.

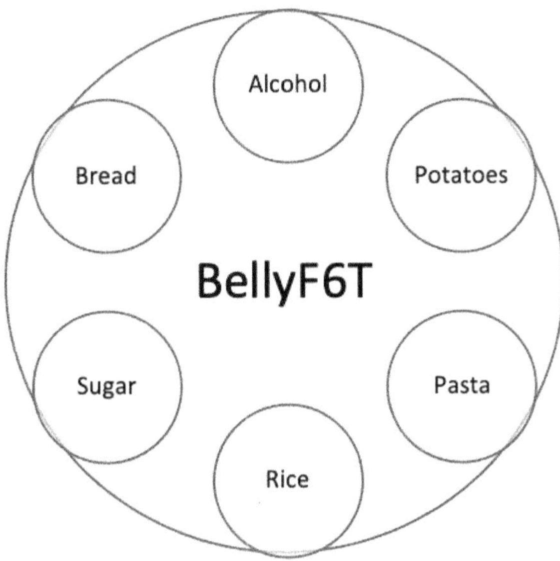

I maintained the process. However, I continued to reduce or eliminate The Belly Fat Six.

The hunger goes. However, when I felt hungry, I realised that this was my body telling me it was using up the fat stores to ensure energy needs are satisfied.

The Belly Fat Six – Part Two

The Next Four Weeks

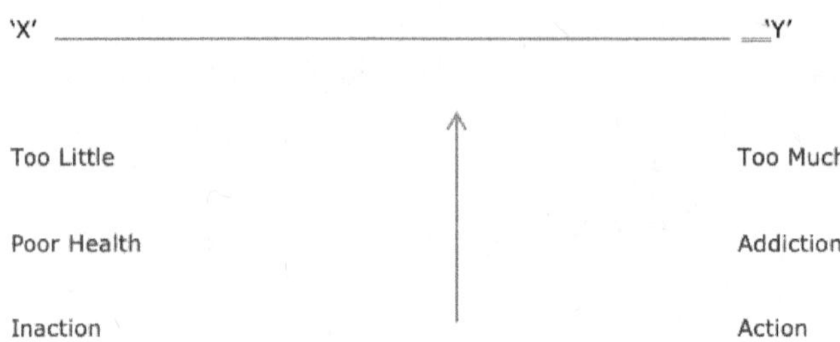

Aim for some action but not too much.

Choose:

- I use my example 'Flexible Daily Intake Plans' as a starting point
- I make my own plans and exclude the Belly Fat Six
- Calorie counting by excluding The Belly Fat Six
- Adding nutritious foods high in minerals and vitamins.

Flexible Daily Intake Plans (Guide Only)

Example 1

- Snack on fruit and vegetables throughout the day.

- Aim for one evening meal of around 1000 to 1500 calories of nutrient dense food sources.

- Incorporate the 8 Superfoods

- Exclude the Belly Fat 6

Example 2

Meal Day	Menu	Calories In		Steps	10363
Anytime	Coffee	20		Calories Out	3321
	Semi Skimmed Milk	224			
Breakfast	Bacon	81		Calories In	1327
	Egg	66			
Morning	Black Olives	144			
Lunch	Cheese slice	50		Deficit	1994
	Sliced Ham	46			
	Coleslaw	98			
	Lettuce	8			
	Tomatoes	16			
	Cucumber	20			
Afternoon				Fat	48
Dinner	Salmon Fillet	200		Protein	22
	Curry Sauce	115			
	Broccoli	34			
Evening	Cornflakes and Milk	205		Carbs	30
Total	Including Snacks	1327			

Example 3

Meal Day	Menu	Calories In		Steps	15561
Anytime	Coffee	20		Calories Out	3515
Breakfast	Eggs	66		Calories In	1287
	Bacon	81			
Morning	Banana	105			
Lunch	Chicken Wraps	155		Deficit	2228
Afternoon	Apple	72		Fat	29%
Dinner	Pasta Bake	559		Protein	20%
	Broccoli	34			
Evening	Cornflakes and milk	205		Carbs	51%
Total	Including Snacks	1287			

Example 4

Meal Day	Menu	Calories In		Steps	8799
Anytime	Coffee	20		Calories Out	3021
Breakfast	Porridge	149			
	Apple	72		Calories In	1321
Morning	Banana	105			
	Black Olives	36			
Lunch	Cheese	236		Deficit	1700
	Crackers	40			
Afternoon	Apple	72		Fat	30%
Dinner	Fajita, Chicken & vegetables	352		Protein	17%
	Broccoli	34			
Evening	Cornflakes & Milk	205		Carbs	53%
Total	Including Snacks	1321			

Example 5

Meal Day	Menu	Calories In		Steps	16212
Anytime	Coffee	20		Calories Out	3714
Breakfast	Banana	105			
	Porridge	149		Calories In	1401
Morning	Black Olives	36			
Lunch	Chicken Burrito	332		Deficit	2313
	Broccoli	34			
Afternoon	Apple	72		Fat	26%
Dinner	Beef Quarter Pound Burger, Steak Cut Chips, Salad	448		Protein	17%
Evening	Cornflakes & Milk	205		Carbs	57%
Total	Including Snacks	1401			

Example 6

Meal Day	Menu	Calories In		Steps	10963
Anytime	Coffee	20		Calories Out	3139
Breakfast	Porridge	149			
	Apple	72		Calories In	1253
Morning	Black Olives	36			
Lunch	Salmon	116		Deficit	1886
	Salad	44			
Afternoon				Fat	32%
Dinner	Chicken Curry, Broccoli	445			
	Poppadom's	34		Protein	23%
		132			
Evening	Cornflakes & Milk	205		Carbs	45%
Total	Including Snacks	1253			

Example 7

Meal Day	Menu	Calories In			
			Steps	16212	
Anytime	Coffee	20	Calories Out	3349	
Breakfast	Porridge	149			
	Apple	72	Calories In	1347	
Morning	Bananas	105			
Lunch	Chips	180	Deficit	2002	
Afternoon			Fat	19%	
	Black Olives	36			
Dinner	Chicken Chow Mein with Rice	580	Protein	18%	
Evening	Cornflakes & Milk	205			
			Carbs	63%	
Total	Including Snacks	1347			

Example 8

Meal Day	Menu	Calories In		Steps	10963
Anytime	Coffee	20		Calories Out	3400
	Semi-skimmed milk	112			
Breakfast	Porridge	149		Calories In	1221
Morning	Black Olives	36			
Lunch	Pork Chops, Carrots and Spinach	525		Deficit	2179
Afternoon				Fat	33%
Dinner	3 Slices Chicken Breast, Mixed Greens, Salad, Coleslaw	174		Protein	34%
Evening	Cornflakes & Milk	205		Carbs	33%
Total	Including Snacks	1221			

Step 2 - Calorie Counting

Or if you prefer: Construct your own 1000 to 1500 calories. Example:

Nutrition Facts Per 100g

Nutrition	Calories	Water	Protein	Carbs	Sugar	Fibre	Fat
Broccoli	31	91	3.7	2.1		2.4	0.8
Leafy Veg	20	92	1.9	1.6		2.6	0.7
Spinach	24	92	2.9	1.3		2.1	0.8
Nuts	622.5		23.3	6.5		5.55	55.8
Oats	140		5	28		4	2.5
Carrots	28		0.7	5.7		2	0.3
Peppers	15		0.8	2.6		1.6	0.3
Olives/ Oil	164	92	1	3.5		3.1	16.2
Spices							
Oranges	37.4	87	1.1	8.5		1.7	0.06
Apples	49		0.35	11.83		1.97	0.1
Bananas	95		1.2	20.09		4.2	0.03
Oily Fish	186		26	0		0	8
Cheese	416		25.4	0.1		0	34.9
Milk (100ml)	48.6		3.4	5.01		0	1.7
Eggs	143		12.5	0		0	10.8
Poultry	195	73%	29.55	0	0	0	10
Beef	217	61%	26.1	0	0	0	11.8
Lamb	258	57%	25.6	0	0	0	16.5
Pork	297	53%	25.7	0	0	0	20.8

Vitamins From a Balanced Diet

Vitamins	Broccoli	Leafy Veg	Spinach	Nuts	Oats	Carrots	Peppers	Olives/Oil	Spices	Oranges	Apples	Banana	Oily Fish	Cheese	Milk	Eggs	Poultry	Beef	Lamb	Pork
A	✓		✓			✓		✓					✓	✓	✓	✓				
B1 Thiamin	✓				✓					✓	✓				✓	✓				✓
B2 Riboflavin	✓		✓		✓						✓		✓	✓	✓	✓				
B3 Niacin				✓				✓					✓		✓	✓	✓	✓	✓	✓
Pantothenic Acid	✓				✓										✓	✓	✓			
B6	✓		✓	✓	✓	✓		✓		✓	✓				✓	✓	✓	✓		✓
B7 Biotin						✓														
Folate Folic	✓	✓	✓	✓						✓					✓					
B12													✓	✓	✓	✓		✓	✓	✓
C	✓	✓	✓								✓	✓			✓					
D													✓		✓	✓				
E	✓		✓	✓				✓							✓	✓				
K	✓	✓	✓	✓		✓		✓				✓			✓	✓				
Calcium	✓	✓	✓	✓				✓			✓		✓	✓	✓					
Iodine													✓							
Iron	✓	✓	✓		✓			✓					✓			✓		✓	✓	✓
Total	11	5	9	6	5	4		7		3	5	2	8	4	13	11	3	4	3	5

Minerals From a Balanced Diet

Minerals	Broccoli	Leafy Veg	Spinach	Nuts	Oats	Carrots	Peppers	Olives/Oil	Spices	Oranges	Apples	Banana	Oily Fish	Cheese	Milk	Eggs	Poultry	Beef	Lamb	Pork
Beta Carotene	✓		✓			✓	✓		✓											
Chromium	✓																			
Cobalt	✓		✓	✓	✓								✓							
Copper			✓	✓	✓			✓				✓				✓				
Magnesium	✓	✓	✓	✓	✓			✓				✓	✓	✓			✓			
Manganese			✓	✓	✓							✓								
Molybdenum	✓		✓	✓	✓															
Phosphorus	✓				✓								✓	✓			✓	✓	✓	✓
Potassium	✓	✓	✓	✓		✓		✓		✓	✓	✓	✓				✓			
Selenium	✓			✓	✓								✓					✓	✓	✓
Salt								✓						✓						
Zinc					✓			✓					✓	✓	✓	✓		✓	✓	✓
Total	8	2	7	7	□	2	1	5	1	1	1	4	6	4	1	2	3	3	3	3

Vitamins & Minerals from a Balanced Diet

Vitamins	Broccoli	Leafy Veg	Spinach	Nuts	Oats	Carrots	Peppers	Olives/Oil	Spices	Oranges	Apples	Banana	Oily Fish	Cheese	Milk	Eggs	Poultry	Beef	Lamb	Pork
A	✓		✓			✓		✓					✓	✓	✓	✓				
B1 Thiamin	✓				✓					✓	✓				✓	✓				✓
B2 Riboflavin	✓		✓		✓						✓		✓	✓	✓	✓				
B3 Niacin				✓				✓					✓		✓	✓	✓	✓	✓	✓
Pantothenic	✓				✓										✓	✓	✓			
B6	✓		✓	✓	✓	✓		✓		✓	✓				✓	✓	✓	✓		✓
B7 Biotin						✓														
Folate Folic	✓	✓	✓	✓						✓					✓					
B12													✓	✓	✓	✓		✓	✓	✓
C	✓	✓	✓					✓		✓		✓			✓					
D													✓		✓	✓				
E	✓		✓	✓				✓							✓	✓				
K	✓	✓	✓	✓		✓		✓			✓				✓	✓				
Calcium	✓	✓	✓	✓				✓			✓		✓	✓	✓					
Iodine													✓							
Iron	✓	✓	✓		✓			✓					✓			✓		✓	✓	✓
Minerals																				
Beta Carotene	✓		✓			✓	✓		✓											
Chromium	✓																			
Cobalt	✓		✓	✓	✓								✓							
Copper			✓	✓	✓			✓				✓				✓				
Magnesium	✓	✓	✓	✓	✓			✓					✓	✓	✓		✓			
Manganese			✓	✓	✓								✓							
Molybdenum	✓		✓	✓	✓															
Phosphorus	✓				✓								✓	✓			✓	✓	✓	✓
Potassium	✓	✓	✓	✓		✓		✓		✓	✓	✓	✓				✓			
Selenium	✓			✓	✓								✓					✓	✓	✓
Salt								✓						✓						
Zinc					✓			✓					✓	✓	✓	✓		✓	✓	✓
Score	19	7	16	13	13	6	1	13	1	4	6	6	14	8	14	13	6	7	6	8

Belly Fat Carbohydrates

Nutritionists and dieticians agree that carbohydrates are our primary source of energy and an essential part of a healthy diet:

I found there are 3 main types of carbohydrates:

1. Sugars
2. Starch
3. Fibre

New Labels

Carbohydrates can be simple or complex and this depends on their chemical structure, and this determines how our body deals with them. There's more confusion as many foods may contain a mixture of simple and complex carbs too. So, to avoid confusion I call them by 3 different labels:

My new carbohydrate labels for my Belly Fat 6 diet.

1. SIMPLEX (instead of simple)
2. **BELLY FAT (my new label)** and
3. COMPLEX

Our body deals with Simplex and Complex carbohydrates in much the same way. These are SMART Carbohydrates.

However, Belly Fat 6 carbohydrates are separated from other carbohydrates because of the separate means in which our body deals with them. The primary reason is that there is no calorific benefit from eating the Belly Fat 6 (and our body knows this)! Not SMART!

Sugar (Belly Fat Carb) V Honey (Simplex Carb)

Honey contains 15 minerals, and 6 vitamins compare this to Sugar that contains 2 minerals and zero vitamins.

BellyF6t

Minerals	Honey	Sugar	Vitamins	Honey	Sugar
Beta Carotene	X	X	A	X	X
Chromium	X	X	B1 Thiamin	YES	X
Cobalt	X	X	B2 Riboflavin	YES	X
Copper	YES	X	B3 Niacin	YES	X
Magnesium	YES	X	Pantothenic Acid	YES	X
Manganese	YES	X	B6	X	X
Molybdenum	X	X	B7 Biotin	X	X
Phosphorus	YES	X	Folate Folic	X	X
Potassium	YES	YES	B12	X	X
Selenium	YES	X	C	X	X
Salt	YES	YES	D	X	X
Zinc	YES	X	E	X	X
Fluoride	YES	X	K	X	X
GI	Low	High	Calcium	YES	X
Calories	64	46	Iodine	X	X
Sub Total	9	2	Iron	YES	X
Total	15	2	Sub Total	6	NONE

On Balance, Sugar, or Honey?

I remember my physics teacher telling the class that if we sweetened everything with honey, we wouldn't have cavities. Apparently, there might be something in this as I found a honey producer advocating that mixing honey with warm water creates a chemical that influences bacteria and prevents plaque as a chemical reaction kind of neutralises the bacteria. Interesting when we consider the difference vitamins and minerals contained in sugar and honey.

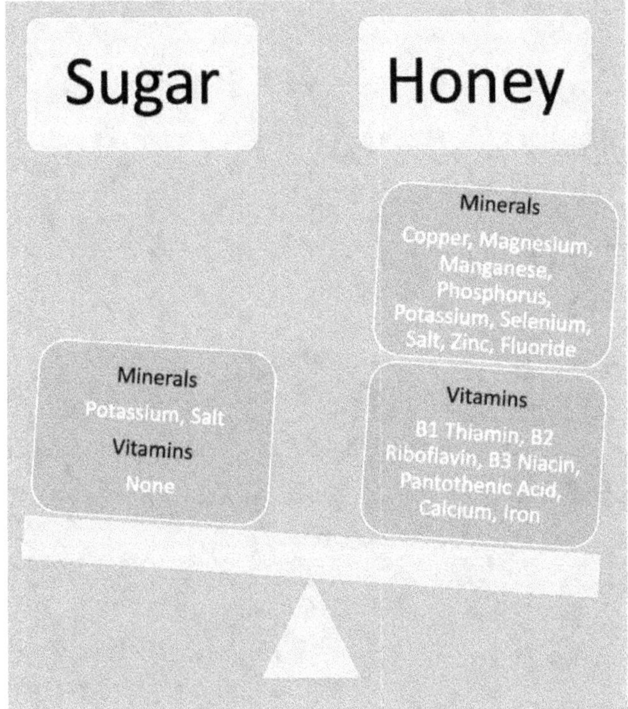
Sugar
Honey
Minerals
Copper, Magnesium, Manganese, Phosphorus, Potassium, Selenium, Salt, Zinc, Fluoride
Minerals
Potassium, Salt
Vitamins
None
Vitamins
B1 Thiamin, B2 Riboflavin, B3 Niacin, Pantothenic Acid, Calcium, Iron

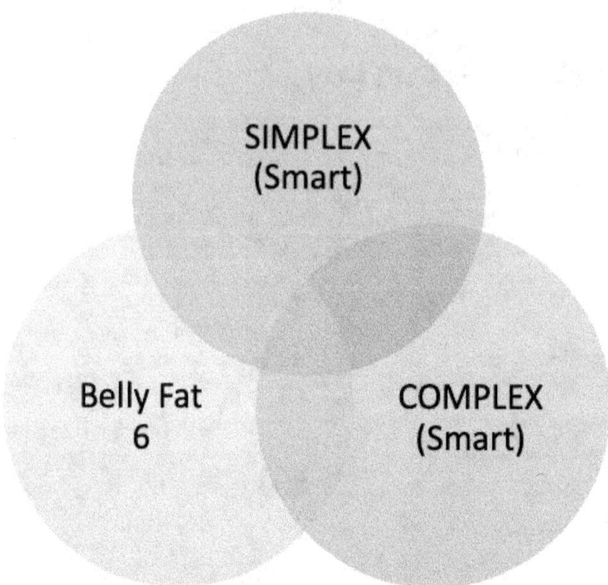

- ❖ Aim for more SIMPLEX,
- ❖ More COMPLEX but
- ❖ We don't want **Belly Fat 6**.

Complex (Smart carbs):

These carbs have longer chains of sugar molecules that mean the body takes longer to break them down. So, these sugars are more difficult to digest and therefore provide a more consistent delivery of energy over a longer period. So, I think I should choose more whole foods for more fibre, vitamins, and minerals than refined or processed foods.

More

- Whole grains
- Barley, Corn
- Black beans, Chickpeas, Lentils, Legumes
- Brown rice
- Vegetables

SIMPLEX – (Smart Carbs)

(Previously Simple)

I label these carbohydrates SIMPLEX to avoid confusion and exclude
Belly Fat Six as Belly Fat Six are not good! Simplex is my third type of
carbohydrate that is 'simple' but the fibre in fruit and vegetables means
they break down like a complex carbohydrate. So, a simplex carb is
really a type of hybrid or crossover carb its main characteristic is that it's
a natural food source.

- Natural sugars   (SIMPLEX)
- Vegetables   (SIMPLEX)
- Fruit   (SIMPLEX)
- Milk   (SIMPLEX)

'Simplex' carbohydrates behave more like Complex carbohydrates and
are smart carbohydrates. But are not like 'Belly Fat 6' carbs (not smart)!

BELLY FAT Six

(Simple / bad Carbs / not smart / The Belly Fat 6)

The Belly Fat Six are all here. All 'Belly Fat Carbs'!

BELLY FAT carbohydrates are easy to digest, they are refined and processed basic sugars and starches and alcohol.

Belly Fat carbs are found in most sweets, chocolates, baked goods, and sugary drinks and alcoholic drinks.

Labelling allows many variations of sugars, and this creates confusion.

Sugar labelling includes:

- Brown sugar
- Corn sweetener
- Corn syrup
- HFCS
- Fructose
- Glucose
- Maltose
- Malt syrup
- Trehalose
- Sucrose
- And many others.

Belly Fat carbohydrates to exclude or limit from our diet include:

The Belly Fat Six

Sugary drinks, Energy drinks, Alcohol, Sweetened tea, or coffee

Sweets, Chocolate, Biscuits, Pastries

Desserts, Ice cream

Carbohydrates, Simplex, Belly Fat 6, Complex

Glycemic Index and Glycemic Load

I don't think adding this type of scientific complexity to a normal person's weight loss programme is worthwhile, I can lose weight by eating less but it is nice to know some of the science behind my foods. I found the glycaemic index (GI) explains how high my blood sugar will rise after eating a specific carbohydrate compared to eating pure sugar.

Basically, the glycaemic load (GL) shows the level of carbohydrate in my food.

- Belly Fat Six foods are high GI and are absorbed quickly.
- Complex and Simplex carbs are Low GI foods digested more slowly.

For those interested, the glycaemic load is calculated by taking the GI and multiplying by the amount of carbohydrate in a normal serving divided by 100.

- LOW GL below 10
- MED GL 11 to 19
- HIGH GL over 20

2 important notes:

- GI & GL is not an indicator of healthy foods. Some high GI foods can be healthy.
- The GI & GL is an unreliable guide when mixing foods or eating on an empty stomach.

Indirect Health Benefits

Excluding The Belly Fat Six led me to believe that I experienced some Indirect Health Benefits for my new lifestyle, and I found examples of other possible associated benefits too, including:

- Irritable Bowel Syndrome and feeling bloated may disappear.
- Avoiding alcohol can mean no more blood in stools
- Reduced inflammation
- Pain in back, knees, wrists, joints may ease
- No more headaches are a good sign
- Feel better, less depression, improved mood
- Improvement in bone health through mineral absorption
- Improve gut health and less likelihood of lactose intolerance
- Skin may improve quickly from eczema or psoriasis
- Increased hair density, and better hair texture
- Nausea may cease

Eat regularly as this helps maintain insulin levels. I also, discovered that fasting encourages sugar spikes.

Summary Table of My Carbohydrates:

My Carbohydrates		
Simplex	**Belly Fat 6**	**Complex**
Easy to digest but slow release of sugar	Easy to digest fast sugar spike	Harder to digest, slow release of sugar
Good Sources: Vegetables Fruit Milk	**Bad Sources:** Brown sugar Corn sweetener Corn syrup HFCS Fructose Glucose Maltose Malt syrup Trehalose Sucrose And many others.	**Good Source:** Whole grains Barley Corn Black beans Chick peas Lentils Legumes Brown rice Vegetables
Include: Broccoli Spinach Leafy Greens Apples Oranges Bananas Milk Honey	**Exclude:** The Belly Fat Six Sugary drinks Energy drinks Alcohol Sweets Chocolate Biscuits Pastries Desserts Ice cream Sweetened tea or coffee	**Include:** Wholefoods

My 8 Superfoods

Because these are nutrient rich and easily digested.

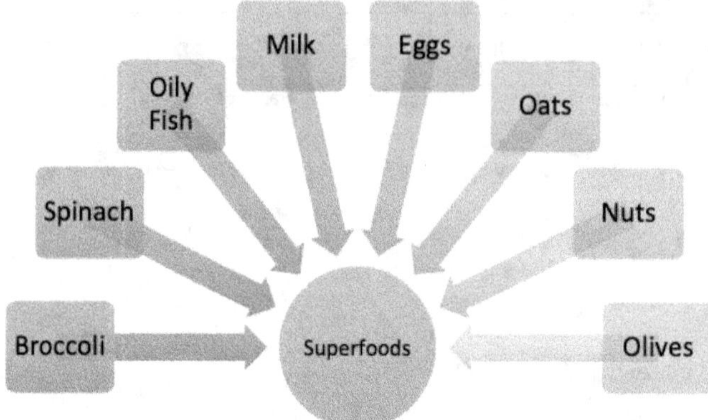

Exercise or Excessive Wear

I'm old and lazy so I walk but don't overdo the exercise myself. I must balance losing weight, getting fit and body damage and time to repair injuries. I found I don't have to exercise to lose weight. Exercise may provide many health benefits. But I found the best way to lose weight is to eat smartly. I aim for exercise/diet balance for my personal needs.

Exercise is great for breathing and healthy heart and lungs, and studies show exercise prevents diabetes and strokes and other ailments. However, exercise can have an adverse effect on other body parts such as knees and hips for example.

There are also many considerations as to the exercise I should be doing. It's common to see warnings about starting to exercise without careful consideration of how fit we really are compared to how fit we think we are. Exercise, exertion, and being unfit are a recipe for complaint, injury, heart attack or worse and can lead to worse circumstances that led to our decision to exercise in the first place.

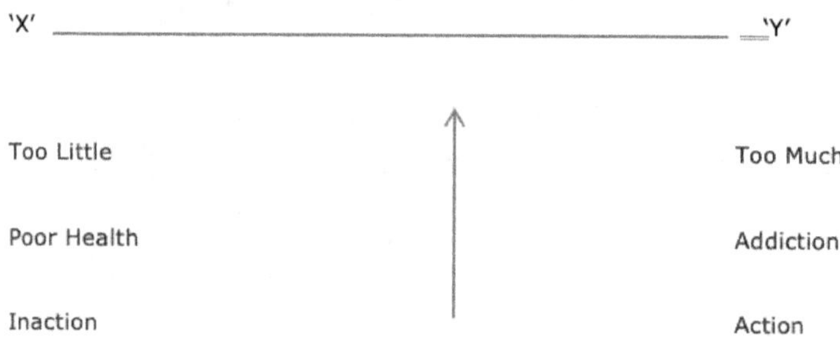

Aim for some action but not too much.

Obesity Battle

As I join the fight against obesity I therefore, consider the fragility of my body. Particularly, my back, neck, knees, ankles, and bones when walking or standing, and never run or jump. I take care lifting, repetition of tasks, I never run and avoid stress, strains, and injuries.

I never realised the many physical activities that have specific injury concerns such as these that I found in my research:

- Tennis elbow
- Golfers groin
- Runner's knee
- Runners claw toe
- Joggers hip
- Jogger's nephritis
- Jumper's ankle

Obviously, the more overweight I am the more risk of injury from exercise. My advice to myself is that if I am overweight, exercise should be light to moderate to reduce the risk of injury from impact on bones and joints and to prevent breathlessness. Exercise should follow weight loss. This warrants the warning that when starting an exercise programme a doctor's advice should be taken.

Viral Risks

More recently highlighted in the 2019 pandemic, there is also a risk of viral infections and other contact diseases, such as:

- Covid19
- Colds and Flu
- Sore throats
- Other respiratory infectious
- Conjunctivitis
- Legionella Disease
- Fungal infections and
- Verrucae

Obviously, the more exercise I do the higher the risk of body damage and accidents. The more contact with others, the higher risk of disease. This has given voice to some medical experts who support quality exercise programmes over quantity.

Some of the medical ethos I found pointed to bones that benefit from exercise in both strength and density. However, the same sources suggest that too much exercise can have the opposite effect and lead to skeletal weaknesses! There's a difference between the genders too, as osteoporosis affects older females where poor diet and menstruation have been issues. Many men in their 50's are at risk from change in lifestyles after years of abuse and on the contrary, football players develop very strong dense ankles and leg bones from running and impact. These two examples demonstrate the need for balance and variety.

My takeaway from exercise is not to overdo it and to choose the right type of exercise for my body and its condition. My doctor advises that swimming is great for stamina and improving respiratory conditions. However, I found squash is much better for building bone density but is straining on the heart. When choose the correct exercise for me, considering lifestyle, Belly Fat Six intake, nutrition, and obesity I will build a stronger mind and body. Poor choices can mean a worsening situation.

With exercise I am better prepared to fight off the big 4 heart attack, stroke, Cancer, and diabetes. My experience found that weight loss through exercise happens, but the other benefits are crucial to my well-being. I concluded that excluding the Belly Fat Six is important as this means my digestive system does less to get more nutrition, and that nutritionists seem to agree that when I lose weight exercise is a means to maintain a healthy weight and lifestyle.

Some Drawbacks	**Some Benefits**
- Time to fit it in - Exercise makes us hungry - Resting after exercise - Wear and tear on joints - Wear and tear on ligaments - Increase chance of accidents - Not a great weight loss method	- Improved blood pressure - Reduced risk of heart disease - Reduced risk of stroke - Reduced risk of diabetes - Reduced risk of Alzheimer's - Reduced risk of dementia - Look great, Feel great - Builds Muscle - Toned body - Healthy mind - Some weight loss - Maintains body weight

Walking

Since I use most of my calories through other activities and normal body functions, I found that gentle exercise is sufficient to change my habitual body weight. Individuals who aim for sporting prowess will have different goals.

Walking uses calories and does not impose the risk that other more vigorous activities such as running might, intensity can be found in hill walking. It's not for me but some people may be more able to exercise in bursts of 15-to-30-minute exertions. But the message is I do what I feel is right for me. But more exercise often means more rest and resting reduces calories used. So, I consider 30 minutes exercise walking my dog and no rest time against going to the gym and 1 hour walk built into a daily routine, (such as a walk to the shop instead of parking the car outside it).

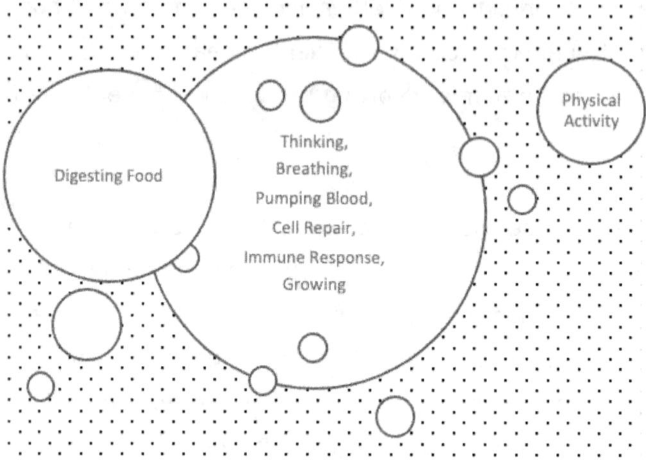

So, surprisingly, my body's burning only around 30% of daily calories through movement. Exercise does not make a huge impact on my calories used!

When I decide to cut the Belly Fat Six, I can choose an exercise regime, or walking routine as well. The choice is mine, it's up to me as an individual but I always track and monitor my progress. Continuing the same routine eating nutritious foods and excluding the Belly Fat Six will trick my body into losing pounds. I will lose around a pound per week but some days I lose a pound per day, but the goal is to keep the lost weight off and not return to old habits as rewards. I made a weight loss of a stone of fat in 14 weeks.

Exercise and Diet, Some Benefits, Yes!

What we eat is more important than what we do, ALWAYS!

The USA and the UK are examples of countries that have issues with food, sugar, marketing, obesity and diabetes as well as other food related concerns. I found studies demonstrating that people all over the world, in cities, jungles, islands, mountains, hot countries and in cold countries use a similar number of calories daily. However, diets vary from the processed foods of sugar and starch to traditional foragers and hunters. Obesity, diabetes, heart disease, joint replacements and other illnesses and issues vary too, especially in countries that have fast food outlets!

What are We Doing?

What we eat versus what we do. It's easy to assume that calorie intake has more effect on obesity than calories out. This statement reflects the many thousands of bodily functions we must do each day to stay alive. Activity levels are about the same too, many people have physical and very active jobs and do not rest from morning to night, but research suggests that obesity remains a bigger issue in the Western World and is growing everywhere in the world.

However, food around the world is very different. Keto diets, Mediterranean diets and low carb diets all have a common theme. These diets tell us what to eat and basically that's whole foods and natural foods and this by conjecture excludes the Belly Fat Six. We are excluding the processed foods such as sugar, rice, pasta, bread and, potatoes and alcohol. Many diets focus on what we should eat, my Belly Fat Six focuses on what I shouldn't eat!

The Belly Fat Six is only different because I am focusing on what makes me fat and what must be excluded to lose weight and to stop adding to the fat that is already there on my belly! I hope this makes sense! I just shift focus to the Belly Fat Six. What to exclude instead of what to include.

Where are these diets?

- o   Sugar Diet?
- o   Rice Diet?
- o   Potato Diet?
- o   Pasta Diet?
- o   Bread Diet?
- o   Alcohol Diet?

These are the foods and drinks that we all cut when we diet. We cut them for a reason. All six cause our belly fat. I call these The Belly Fat Six and cutting these 6 items from our diets alone will influence our obesity levels. The focus must be here. Many countries around the world do not naturally include these foods in their diet, some countries exclude alcohol and while some countries have meat, fish, or vegetable-based diets it is largely considered from my research that it's The Belly Fat Six that causes obesity and other health problems.

So, around the world we have the same daily calories out varying calories in, but the world's population have different diets. One common thing is that, once I have reached a maximum weight my body seems to always try to return to this maximum weight, do people really have an obesity memory? Is this the reason I find it extremely difficult to lose weight because of the habits I have built into my natural rhythm. Overcoming the circadian fat memory will take a determined focus as there are many obstacles to overcome. Knowledge is the key to change, knowing what to do, how to do it and being prepared all help to change habits.

Health and Immunity

I'm going off track a little because in the research I found interesting points about food, immunity, and nutrition as I wanted to be healthy as well as lose a few pounds. So, I've included a few random interesting points from my research.

A healthy immune system helps me to provide a response to viral infections and bacteria that cause our bodies harm. I found T Cells and B Cells are an important part of staying healthy. Simply put, these important cells are produced in our bones and bone marrow and trained in our thymus gland to either defend the body from attack or kill the invading infections.

The problem for our immune systems is once we reach adolescence the thymus gland has mostly done its job. Thereafter, the thymus gland starts to become fatty tissue and by the age of 75 for most people the thymus gland is a ball of fat, a natural ageing process. It has been thought the thymus gland cannot be stimulated but research in the USA regarding HIV found that it's possible the thymus gland could be stimulated. Vitamin A is found to stimulate T Cell response while Vitamin C increases the number of T Cells while also helping to condition the size and weight of the thymus. So, how might our diet help maintain or stimulate our thymus gland?

Key foods for a healthy immune response using the Belly Fat 6 analysis are:

- Oily Fish - 6
- Broccoli - 5
- Milk - 5
- Honey - 4
- Olives / Olive Oil - 4

Minerals & Vitamins	Broccoli	Leafy Veg	Spinach	Nuts	Oats	Carrots	Honey	Olives/Oil	Spices	Oranges	Apples	Banana	Oily Fish	Cheese	Milk	Eggs	Poultry	Beef	Lamb	Pork
Cell Production																				
D													✓		✓	✓				
Calcium	✓	✓	✓	✓			✓	✓			✓		✓	✓	✓					
Phosphorus	✓				✓		✓						✓	✓			✓	✓	✓	✓
Stimulate Thymus Gland																				
A	✓		✓			✓		✓					✓	✓	✓	✓				
C	✓	✓	✓					✓		✓		✓			✓					
Selenium	✓			✓	✓		✓						✓					✓	✓	✓
Zinc					✓		✓	✓					✓	✓	✓	✓		✓	✓	✓
Total	5	2	3	2	3	2	4	4	0	1	1	1	6	4	5	3	1	3	3	3

Applying the Belly Fat 6 analysis this is what we found:

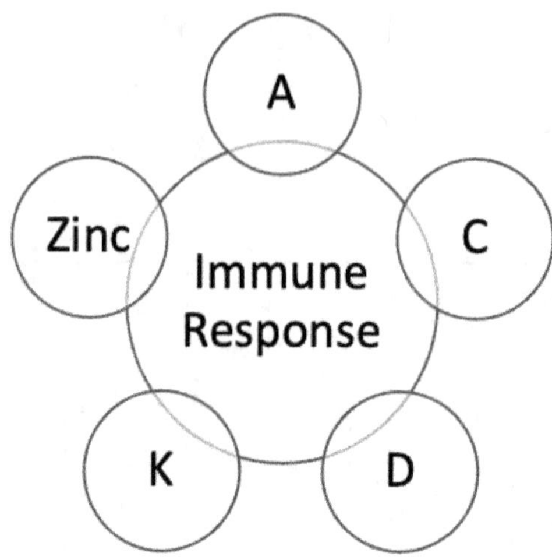

Not surprisingly Mediterranean perhaps! Ancient Rome! Fish, vegetables, and cheese was a part of the Roman diet. Turns out the thymus gland in modern times has been discarded as a not so important body part (even though it is situated near to the heart).

However, it seems, the T Cells that are much needed to fight off infections are really named thymus cells in the medical world! The importance is not new, and I found that in ancient times the Romans regarded the thymus as the body's soul and spirit.

Apparently, that empty feeling, we get above the sternum when we are stressed or upset is also the place, where we feel joy and happiness. Right next to and slightly above the heart the thymus stores our T Cells ready for deployment against viral and bacterial infections!

I found the general medical position is that when people reach adolescence the thymus has done its job, trained our T Cells and begun to deplete until by the age of 65 to 75 the thymus is nothing more than a ball of gristly fat. However, I found that not all people agree with this and HIV research in the USA is reported as promising regarding the stimulation of the thymus and alternative medicine such as acupuncture believe the thymus may just require unblocking. This is an area for others to research and provide answers.

Immune Response

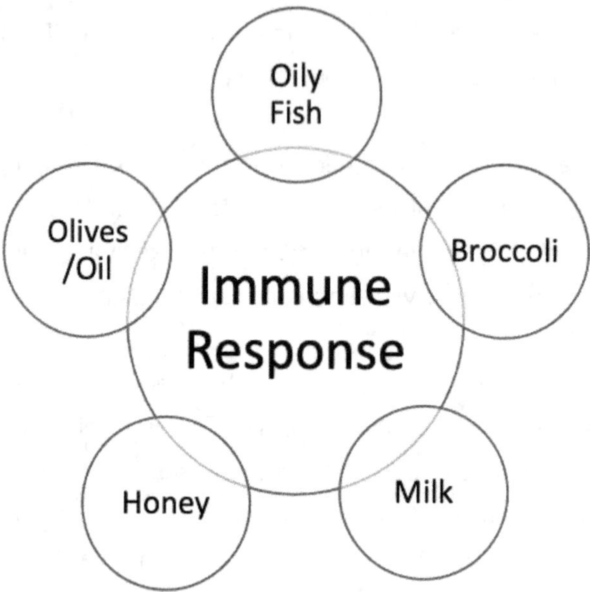

Therefore, this important body part may not be receiving the attention it really deserves and may require much more scientific explanation. For example, I found that only since the 1960's has there been any progress in the importance of the thymus and while some scientific leaps have been made it seems that massive investment during the 2019 pandemic that has highlighted vitamins A, C, D and K and zinc as vital for cell development, thymic stimulation, and immune response.

Why Being Fit and Healthy Is Important to me

- Lower triglycerides
- Lower blood pressure
- Lower risk of diabetes
- Lower risk of Alzheimer's
- Lower risk of dementia
- Lower risk of some cancers

Back on Track

I found there are many benefits attributed to exercise however significant weight loss may not be one of them. I found exercise does influence weight loss but much less than I expected but I did feel good.

I found that activity only accounts for around 10% to 30% of calories I use each day. Most calories are burned through the thousands of bodily functions I must do daily to exist and the digestion of food.

I'm now concerned that even after intense physical activity I may eat the calories I burned and reduce my activity to rest and recover.

The research demonstrates 3 dynamics to energy expenditure:

1. Energy used for essential body functions. 60 to 80%

2. Energy used to break down food. 10 to 40% and

3. Energy used in physical activity. 10 to 30%

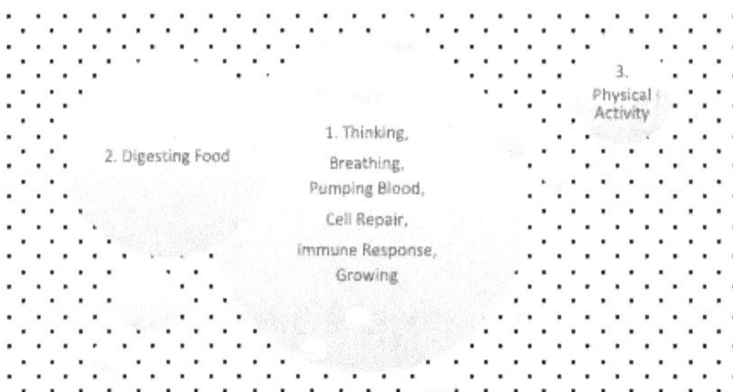

Control

We have little control over the energy expended through our essential body functions. I think we can possibly control our food intake and how our body needs to respond to digest the types of food we eat by eating the 8 superfoods and excluding the Belly Fat Six. Physical activity is both controlled and uncontrolled, for example movement associated with essential body functions is largely uncontrolled but going to work, the gym or driving the car are my personal choices. So, while exercise contributes to my weight loss, my diet and my essential body functions are more influential to my body weight fluctuations. However, I can influence how hard my works by the quality of the food I choose to eat as some foods are more nutritious and more easily digested than others.

I think it's difficult to create a calorie deficit with exercise alone.

I found that nutritionists are aware that exercise alone is not a very useful means of achieving weight loss. Therefore, I monitor and review my weight regularly to help me stay on track.

For example: a 200-pound me exercises 4 hours per week and consumes my normal calorific intake. Over a month I expect a weight loss of 4 to 6 pounds. However, any increase in calories, rest, or relaxation to recover from the added exercise, weight lost could be less than 4 pounds for a month's exercise.

However, I found some experts agree that, maintaining weight loss through exercise requires calorie control and tracking, so monitoring and review helps.

Excluding The Belly Fat Six could mean losing and additional 2 LB's per week, around 8 pounds per month, so a total of exercise and excluding The Belly Fat Six equals a 12-pound weight loss. Because I am excluding the food that makes me fat in the first place!

A big drawback is that exercise makes me feel good and deserving of a reward and I am also hungrier than I would normally be and meaning I probably consume more calories than I lost exercising. I do some activity then replace the calories in one rewarding meal, then rest! I eat Belly Fat 6 and make my body work harder for nothing. And other effects of exercise mean I drive the car instead of walking, move less because of exhaustion or have a treat to reward myself for hard work that might include a takeaway and alcohol. Not anymore!

The Exercise Jeopardy

Exercise makes me hungry and is therefore, directly related to how much I eat, how exhausted I get and how long my recovery takes.

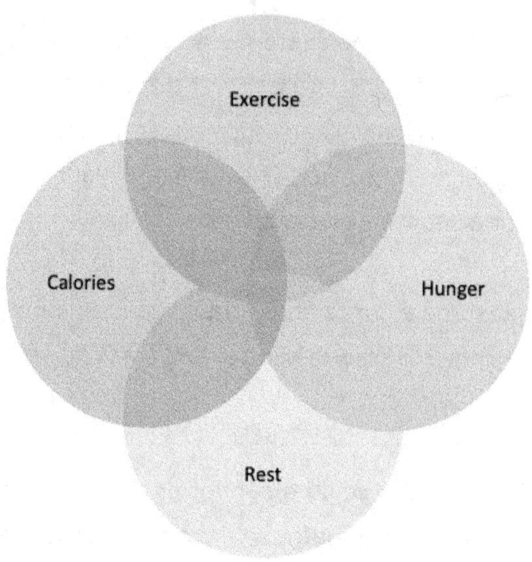

Starvation Mode, An Excuse for not following the plan!

I hear people talking about not losing weight because our bodies go into survival mode. There must be a reason for this. I think that we may not be eating less than we think or creating a calorie deficit as its logically impossible to not lose weight when there is a calorie deficit.

There is a theory I found in my research called 'metabolic compensation' where our bodies make allowances for our activity. This will include exercise and all the other natural body functions such as pumping blood and digesting food. My research found that for some people, exercise may result in fewer calories burned compared to what was expected to burn. This means a workout may not be the most efficient means of weight loss, but it obviously has other benefits, for example heart health.

I find the best way for me is to steer clear of scientific information and focus on the exclusion of the Belly Fat Six, that's much simpler for me!

Metabolic Compensation could be a natural survival mode that people talk about or related to being fitter, but it maybe explains exercise as a weight loss activity may peak for some people at some stage. Or at least that's what some people think. Maybe in reality we are eating more because exercise makes us hungrier. (Or we are subject to food, diet, exercise, and healthy body advertising). Meaning we may not benefit as we think from our activities. Therefore, I focus attention on monitoring what I eat and what I do and compare to the results I achieve. I also found articles that mention that survival mode may also continue to affect calories in and out even if we regain the weight we have lost. A minefield of diet complexity.

This implies that I may continue to conserve my fat stores because I have been forcing my body into survival mode (or I may think this is an extreme case of circadian rhythm exhaustion). In any event, this seems unhealthy, and could cause exercise addiction or weight loss depression. When I hear people saying that they think they need 'a pick me up', this is what I think of!

I think we should aim for balance, as both extremes, depression, and addiction, will affect body and mind.

Too Little
Attention

Too Much
Attention

I found that the survival mode is often referred to when people are having difficulty shifting weight despite exercising. The media makes me assume our bodies may be conserving energy for some future energy needs. We don't know why, who or how long it will continue after exercise or when our circadian rhythm returns to normal. However, the chances are always that, what we disrupt we can repair. We can reset the body clock through focus on healthy lifestyle choices, excluding The Belly Fat Six, eliminating stress and balanced exercise and nutrition.

Too Much Exercise & Calorific Stagnation!

Exercise v Energy Theory

1. The more we exercise the more energy we burn
2. The more we exercise the more our body will conserve energy by compensating on physiological needs.
3. Exercise may therefore peak.

Some research I found, suggests that some people may 'hit a wall' around exercise burning 180 to 220 calories per day, there is a limit to how many calories our bodies will burn in a day, but this is just a theory, or is it? One professor suggested to me that there is thinking around what we eat doesn't matter providing we get our daily calories. I immediately cross reference this thinking with the need to categorise carbohydrates with my 3 labels as my body treats different food sources in different ways.

Diet, Exercise and Misinformation

Exercise, sugar free, light, low fat, fat free, are all growth industries. Designed to keep us fit and healthy. What I've noticed since the 70's and 80's is that people are fatter? Sports injuries have increased and operations for knees and hips were unheard of!

- Many institutions have an interest in cheap food, as there are so many people to feed every day.
- Food producers are in the business of making money from our glut.
- Sports outfitters rely on people wanting to lose weight and get fit.
- There is also a host of diet programs, books, and clubs to help us lose the pounds we bought at the supermarket too.
- I hope The Belly Fat 6 is a bit more focused on health and weight.
- I'm also intrigued at the change in shape of second year university students. Is twenty an age of weight gain?

We are all becoming more obese not just because we are eating more but specifically because we eat The Belly Fat Six. And are encouraged to eat The Belly Fat Six too as we are saturated with advertising and attractive packaging that promote foods that have no or low nutritional value. It is very difficult to wade through all the information about food, diet, vitamins, minerals, calories, nutrition and all the medical effects, most people do not have this level of knowledge and I don't have the time to find the answers either, relying on unchallenged experts for advice.

There are many companies that have business interests based on their customers becoming at risk to heart disease, stroke, diabetes, Alzheimer's, dementia, high blood pressure and a host of cancers. Also, the environmental damage caused by these companies and their packaging doubly affects our well-being too. And, of course they will tell their customers they need to exercise more!

I think people are at a danger of losing all sense toward food, diet, exercise, and obesity when without doubt it's too much of the wrong food that's making the world fat, too much Belly Fat 6. Consumers are a dream for food suppliers who want us to eat more and more. Therefore, dieting becomes a positive source of revenue, and a food industry expands. So do our waistlines!

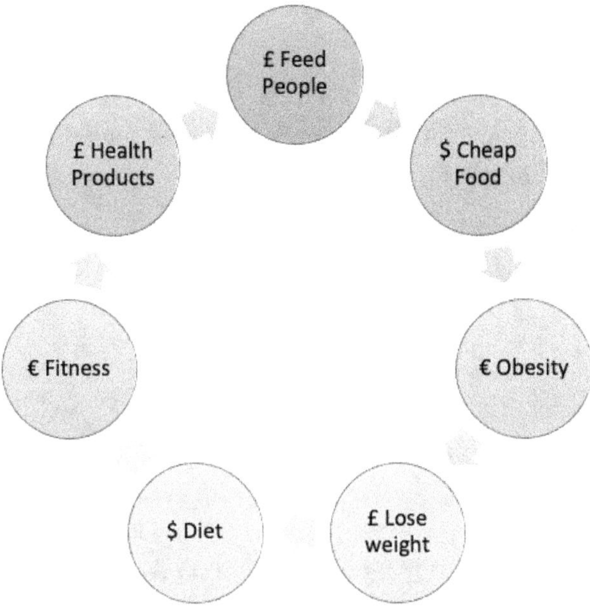

Exercise is essential for mind and body well-being but doubtful it's best for weight-loss. Exercise makes us hungry!

So, what works for weight loss?

The answer for me is:

- Eating less! Do this by eating nutritious food over junk food.
- Eating the right foods, the 8 Superfoods.
- Excluding The Belly Fat 6.
- Moderate exercise

Most energy 60% is used for bodily functions. People can't control such functions as pumping blood.

20% to 40% of our energy used digesting our food.
10% to 30% of calories used for movement, including exercise.

We use more calories pumping blood than pumping iron

Summary:

Step 1

- Prepare for the project physically and mentally
- Exclude The Belly Fat Six
- Calorie intake for a normal adult.
- Increase daily steps by walking outdoors. I don't run.
- If I feel I need more intensity, then I walk up hills.
- Eat nutrition dense foods, eat the 8 superfoods
- Snack on fruit and vegetables
- Plenty of water
- Weigh daily and calculate BMI

Note:

When I exclude the Belly Fat Six, I noticed I have lots of options to eat more food, more vitamins and more minerals and less calories!

This is because the Belly Fat Six is calorie intensive and simply a waste of calories, empty calories.

Then:

Step 2

- Cut calorific intake to 1000 to 1500 calories per day
- Aim for reduced calorie intake (you should see results in the first few days
- Exclude Belly Fat 6 (Restrict Negative vitamin/mineral intake)
- Increase intake of foods high in Vitamin/Mineral
- Walk (Exercise regularly for health but not for weight loss)
- After 4 weeks reduced calories, I returned to my normal adult calorific intake

- One important thing to remember is to eat healthily and limit negative foods, that's the Belly Fat 6
- Exercise and diet have benefits,
- However, exercise alone makes only a marginal difference
- It's important not to count additional calories burned through exercising as an extra food bonus
- After one month of reduced calories, I returned to normal calorie intake for an adult for 6 weeks before repeating the reduced 1500 calories intake.

Actual Results

My results showed a weight loss of a stone in 2 months. From 15 stone to 14 stone and note the weight records varied up and down daily but overall, the trend was to lose weight over the 8 weeks.

Date	Weight	BMI
05/07	14 st 0 lbs	27.4% fat
04/07	14 st 4 lbs	27.9% fat
03/07	14 st 6 lbs	28.2% fat
02/07	14 st 4 lbs	27.9% fat
01/07	14 st 5 lbs	28.1% fat
30/06	14 st 5 lbs	28.1% fat
29/06	14 st 5 lbs	28.1% fat
19/06	14 st 7 lbs	28.2% fat
17/06	14 st 6 lbs	28.2% fat
16/06	14 st 6 lbs	28.2% fat
15/06	14 st 6 lbs	28.2% fat
14/06	·14 st 8 lbs	28.6% fat
13/06	14 st 6 lbs	28.2% fat
12/06	14 st 7 lbs	28.4% fat
11/06	14 st 9 lbs	28.7% fat
10/06	14 st 10 lbs	28.8% fat
23/05	14 st 11 lbs	28.9% fat
13/05	14 st 12 lbs	29.1% fat
10/05	14 st 11 lbs	28.9% fat
08/05	15 st 0 lbs	29.4% fat

Finally, what I eat and what I do

How I use my daily calories.

- Natural body functions calorific output
- Digestion of food
- Physical activity

1. I use calories just being alive.
2. I often exhaust myself by eating hard to digest foods.
3. When I eat easily digestible foods, natural foods, nothing processed, I get more of what my body needs to survive from fewer foods, and this means my body doesn't work so hard digesting foods that are low in nutrients. For example, pound for pound broccoli has many more vitamins and minerals required for healthy lifestyles than for example a cup cake.
4. Treat physical activity as a means of providing health benefits for body and mind and not as a weight loss activity. Exercise helps protect against heart attack, stroke, and diabetes, helps me feel good, benefits my mental health, tones my body and as a by-product of exercise I may lose weight (when I have a calorie deficit)!

Wrapping Up the Belly Fat Six

Step 1: Eat Normally
- Adult Woman 1800 calories
- Adult Man 2300 calories
- Exclude the Belly Fat Six

Walk
- Outside
- 10,000 steps per day

Nutrients
- Eat Vitamin rich foods
- Eat Mineral rich foods

Superfoods
- 8 Superfoods, Fruit
- Include these in your diet

The BellyFat6
- Step 1: Reduce intake of Belly Fat 6
- Step 2: Then Eliminate Belly Fat 6

Step 2: When ready
- Reduce Calories to 1500 per day
- Eliminate BellyFat6, eat nutrient dense foods
- Continue to walk 10,000 steps per day

Tracking
- Weigh Daily
- Record BMI daily

Reduced Calories Diet
- Maximum 4 weeks
- Then return to Step 1

2 Recipe Ideas

Home-made vegetable soup:

Ingredients:

Butternut Squash
Carrots
White Onion
Stock cube (optional)

Method:

Chop squash, carrots, and onion
Place in a large saucepan with stock cube
Cover with water
Bring to boil and simmer until cooked
Liquidise

Cornflour Curry Sauce:

Ingredients

1 tablespoon of cornflour

3 tablespoons curry powder (add to suit taste)

1 onion

1 or 2 apples

1 pint of water

Stock cube (Optional)

Method:

Chop onion and apple

Add to pan and cover with 1 pint of water

Bring to boil and simmer until cooked

Add the curry powder and reduce heat

Mix cornflour with a little cold water

Bring the pan back to the boil

Add the cornflour/water mixture and stir while thickening

Simmer 10 Minutes

Bibliography:

Matthew Edmund MD, The Power of Rest, 2010

Dr Robert Lustig, Fat Chance 2012

Jeanette P Moreno, Potential circadian and circannual rhythm contributions to the obesity epidemic in elementary school age children, pdf, 2019

Dr Satchin Panda, The Circadian Code: Lose weight, supercharge your energy and sleep well every night 2018

Yudkin, John. Pure, White and Deadly 1972

Internet Links:

Chloe Bennett, Circadian Rhythm and Weight Loss
https://www.google.co.uk/amp/s/www.news-medical.net/amp/health/Circadian-Rhythm-and-Weight-Loss.aspx

Why we shouldn't exercise to lose weight. Julia Belluz and Javier Zarracina
https://www.vox.com/2016/4/28/11518804/weight-loss-exercise-myth-burn-calories

Fish Calories and Nutrition Facts: The Best Fish to Lose Weight and Improve Health By Malia Frey
https://www.verywellfit.com/the-best-fish-to-lose-weight-3495772

Circadian rhythms and exercise — re-setting the clock in metabolic disease. Brendan M. Gabriel & Juleen R. Zierath
https://www.nature.com/articles/s41574-018-0150-x

What Does It Mean to Eat According to Your Bio-Circadian Rhythm? Gina Diamond 2020
https://www.ecoparent.ca/eco-food/bio-circadian-rhythm-diet-eating

9 Proven Ways to Fix The Hormones That Control Your Weight, Franziska Spritzler, RD, CDE

https://www.healthline.com/nutrition/9-fixes-for-weight-hormones

When you eat can be just as important as what you eat. Emily Manoogian, https://ideas.ted.com/when-you-eat-can-be-just-as-important-as-what-you-eat/amp/

Knowing When To Hibernate (and When To Wake Up), Ed Grabianowski, https://animals.howstuffworks.com/animal-facts/hibernation2.htm

https://www.bbc.co.uk/news/health-63134505 BBC News: Eating Within Set Times Good For Shift Workers

How Do You Tell the Difference Between Good and Bad Carbohydrates? Diana Rodriguez
https://www.everydayhealth.com/diet-nutrition/diet/good-carbs-bad-carbs/

Foods with The Highest Water Content
https://greenblender.com/smoothies/2683/foods-with-the-highest-water-content

Water in Broccoli
http://www.dietandfitnesstoday.com/water-in-broccoli.php

Oatmeal Nutrition and Facts
https://www.verywellfit.com/oats-nutrition-facts-calories-and-health-benefits-4118577#oatmeal-nutrition-facts

6 Simple Ways to Lose Belly Fat, Based on Science, Kris Gunnars 2020
https://www.healthline.com/nutrition/6-proven-ways-to-lose-belly-fat

20 Common Reasons Why You're Not Losing Weight By Kris Gunnars, BSc 2018
https://www.healthline.com/nutrition/20-reasons-you-are-not-losing-weight

Calorie Counter for U.K. Foods
https://www.weightlossresources.co.uk/calories/calorie_counter.htm

Nutritional Facts
https://www.myfitnesspal.com/food/calories/cornflour-4-tsp-539331402

Food Calorie List

https://www.uncledavesenterprise.com/file/health/Food%20Calories%20List.pdf

Why Diets Don't Work... and What Does
For lifelong weight loss, lose the diet. Meg Selig
https://www.google.co.uk/amp/s/www.psychologytoday.com/gb/blog/changepower/201010/why-diets-dont-work-and-what-does%3famp

https://www.ncbi.nlm.nih.gov/pmc/articles/PMC2738337/

https://purerecoveryca.com/4-benefits-of-quitting-sugar-7-ways-its-similar-to-drugs/

https://www.google.co.uk/search?q=benefits+of+quitting+pasta&ie=UTF-8&oe=UTF-8&hl=en-gb&client=safari

https://www.dummies.com/article/body-mind-spirit/physical-health-well-being/diet-nutrition/wheat-free/10-benefits-of-living-wheat-free-154230/

https://www.google.co.uk/search?q=benefits+of+not+eating+potatoes&ie=UTF-8&oe=UTF-8&hl=en-gb&client=safari

https://www.priorygroup.com/blog/benefits-of-giving-up-alcohol-for-a-month

Honey Teeth Benefits https://mypenndentist.org/dental-tips/2021/09/07/does-honey-rot-your-teeth/

***Before starting any weight loss or exercise programme you should consult your doctor first.**

Link to Google Drive Belly Fat Six A4 Files Pdf:

https://drive.google.com/drive/folders/1PB97-dcmnSTrVa--ZnD2BNlInA-qv0Be?usp=sharing

Clargaux@gmail.com

The Belly Fat Six

6 Belly Fat Carbs to Ditch

- Sugar
- Pasta
- Potatoes
- Rice
- Alcohol
- Bread

D.I.E.T.

- D   Ditch Belly Fat Carbohydrates
- I   Invest in YOU
- E   Eat Nutritious Dense Foods
- T   Track your progress daily

The 8 Superfoods

Broccoli, Spinach, Oily Fish, Milk

- Broccoli: Vitamin A, B1, B2 Riboflavin, Pantothenic Acid, B6, Folate/Folic Acid, C, E, K, Calcium, Iron, Beta Carotene, Chromium, Cobalt, Magnesium, Molybdenum, Phosphorous, Potassium,

- Spinach: Vitamin A, B2 Riboflavin, B6, Folate/Folic Acid, C, E, K, Calcium, Iron, Beta Carotene, Cobalt, Copper, Magnesium, Manganese, Molybdenum, Potassium

- Oily Fish: Vitamin A, B2 Riboflavin, B3 Niacin, B12, Calcium, Magnesium, Phosphorous, Potassium, Selenium, Zinc

- Milk: Vitamin A, B1 Thiamin, B2 Riboflavin, B3 Niacin, Pantothenic Acid, B6, Folate/Folic Acid, B12, C, D, E, K, Calcium, Zinc

Eggs, Oats, Nuts, Olives

- Eggs: Vitamin A, B1 Thiamin, B2 Riboflavin, B3 Niacin, Pantothenic Acid, B6, B12, D, E, K, Iron, Copper, Zinc

- Oats: B1 Thiamin, B2 Riboflavin, Pantothenic Acid, B6, Iron, Cobalt, Copper, Magnesium, Manganese, Molybdenum, Phosphorous, Selenium, Zinc

- Nuts: B3 Niacin, B6, Folate/Folic Acid, E, K, Calcium, Cobalt, Copper, Magnesium, Manganese, Molybdenum, Potassium, Selenium

- Olives: Vitamin A, B3 Niacin, B6, C, E, K, Calcium, Iron, Copper, Magnesium, Potassium, Salt, Zinc

BELLYF6T

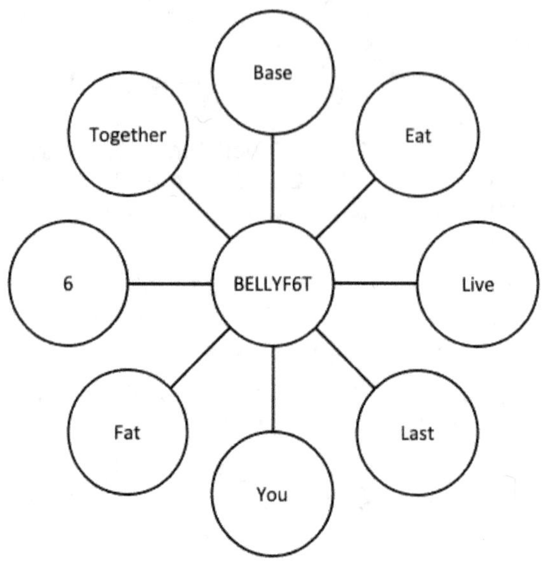

Base	Record starting point!
Eat	Eat well and change what I eat
Live	Have a fun, healthy life with easy nutrition
Last	An eating system to last my lifetime
You	This is all about me, my diet, my life
Fat	Not all fats are bad, Belly fat is.
6	Don't eat Belly Fat carbs, that's the BellyF6t
Team	We are all in this together, spread the word

About The Belly Fat Six

There are knowledge gaps in our nutrition. We believe there are two types of carbohydrates! There are in fact three types of carbohydrates.

New Labels: We are familiar with two types of carbohydrates, complex and simplex that are applied to our food resources because these carbohydrates perform in a particular way.

However, we have allowed some food types to be categorised as simple carbohydrates when these food types, really don't fit into the normal simple and complex categories. Therefore, for the purpose of Belly Fat Six we have assigned new labels for carbohydrates that are more specific terms than simple and complex and separate out the foods that make us fat and prevent weight loss, these foods are the Belly Fat Six and form my new category of carbohydrates. The term Simple carbohydrate has also been redefined. These new labels designed because of this research and for the easy recognition of the Belly Fat Six help me immediately distinguish nutritious and not so nutritious foods!

Identifying nutritious foods that reduced stresses on my body's digestion system means that I can eat less, be healthier, less exhausted and spend less time being nutritionally anxious about myself.

The Belly Fat Six is not so revolutionary as being an alternative way to look at the same old dietary problems. However, the alternative way, is for me, a superior means of analysis. The adage is that, when we keep doing the same things we can expect to be, at best, in the same position. Therefore, the Belly Fat Six is a new lifestyle change that moves forward our thinking by injecting change into industrial norms. The change is the way the Belly Fat Six categorises carbohydrates. See for yourself!

At first, when I tried to lose weight, I increased my weight! However, I was able to initiate results purely by accident and over the course of a couple of months I lost a stone in weight. I then discovered how to lose weight and that I needed to change my eating habits forever. Once we know how to do something it's easier to get results.

I had dived into a diet without preparing nor understanding that losing weight is a massive undertaking. I fell into the trap of clearing the fridge on the eve of my diet commencing, not a good start! This is the sign of an immediate failure and there are many better ways to prepare for the lifestyle change. After making the decision to change the experience should be a pleasant one, and this is how I began the Belly Fat Six. Clear simple explanations so I understand what makes me fat and what happens when I exclude fat producing foods. A few steps to take and preparing the body and mind for success, are all key.

- Reset our body clock and eliminate stress.
- Understand our journeys and the importance of preparation and natural solutions.
- A no nonsense insight and a valuable alternative lifestyle approach.
- New labels that clearly identify empty calories.

When I understood how to achieve weight loss and after having the practical experience, I decided to share my experiences with a little research added into the mix. To help explain the journey and the methods I used, I have made some important and practical weight loss tools that may be useful. It's as easy as riding a bike and once you know how to ride a bike, you never forget. This is how to cement the weight loss technique into my lifestyle choices. But anyone can do this, it's very simple, very natural and it does not require hard work and the technique is easy to remember. Why over-complicate?